The Skidmore-Roth Outline Series:
GERIATRIC NURSING

A SKIDMORE-ROTH PUBLICATION

SR
PUBLISHING

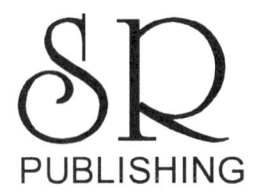

Series Editor: Sheila Passin-Swall
Cover Design: Veronica Burnett
Typesetting: Business Support Centre

Copyright 1996 by Skidmore-Roth Publishing, Inc. All rights reserved. No part of this book may be copied or transmitted in any form or by any means without written permission of the publisher.

Notice: The author and the publisher of this volume have taken care to make certain that all information is correct and compatible with the standards generally accepted at the time of publication.

Voss-Morice, Sidney
The Skidmore-Roth Outline Series: Geriatric Nursing/Sidney Voss-Morice

1. Nursing-Handbooks, Manuals
2. Medical-Handbooks, Manuals

SKIDMORE-ROTH PUBLISHING, INC.
2620 S. Parker Rd., Ste. 147
Aurora, CO 80014
1 (800) 825-3150

Dedication

I would like to dedicate this book to the four pillars in my life - Ginger, Gayle, Curt and Chris.

Contributing Authors

Peggy Szwabo, P.hD., R.N., M.S.W
St. Louis University
Department of Gero-Psychiatry

Helen Lach, R.N., M.S.N.
Program on Aging
Jewish Hospital
St. Louis, MO

Nan Roberts, R.N., M.S.N.
Clinical Nurse Specialist
St. Joseph Home Care
St. Louis, MO

Candy Ross, R.N., M.S.N.
St. Louis University
School of Nursing

TABLE OF CONTENTS

UNIT 1
Profile of the Elderly in America 1

Chapter 1
Aging 2

Chapter 2
Who are the Elderly 33

Chapter 3
The Healthy Older American: Assessment of
the Geriatric Client 65

Chapter 4
Mental Health of the Elderly 120

Chapter 5
The High Risk Profile 147

UNIT 2
The Elderly American: Less than
Optimal Health 173

Chapter 1
Ethical Dilemmas 174

Chapter 2
The Hospitalized Elderly 184

Chapter 3
Home Health Care for the Elderly Client 220

UNIT 3
The Elderly Individual: Legal and Social Issues **239**

Chapter 1
Politics of Aging 240

Chapter 2
A View From the Top 265

Unit 1

Profile of the Elderly American

Unit 1 - Chapter 1

Where Are The Elderly?

Imagine for just a minute what it must be like to be very old today; waking up and not being able to see the time on the bedside clock without putting on your glasses; listening to sounds from your spouse in the same room speaking to you, but hearing only muffled tones; not being able to stand erect because of the osteoporotic changes in your back; not feeling the full sensation of the floor beneath your feet as you begin that long walk to the bathroom.

Though these are the grim realities of the aging process, they are not limitations of very active, very enthusiastic older Americans who present themselves to the Health Care Professionals' door every day, looking for answers to their aches, their pains, and their frustrations.

For every older adult in the hospital or nursing home, there are thousands more in the community utilizing the many resources now available. Their purpose in life has changed over the life-span, but their need for quality of care and concern has not. Are we prepared to meet these needs, create new services and respond in a way which is not only beneficial to them, but also within the realm of what is economically and ethically feasible? Can the health care industry of the 1990's develop a system that will be effective and responsive to the needs of the 'Baby Boomers' of the twenty first century?

There is a tendency for all of society to pin labels on subgroups of the population. As health care professionals, we are keenly aware that there is no discrimination when it comes to disease processes and the effects of unhealthy living. Young and old alike are suffering all over the world with diseases that researchers have yet to conquer. The aged today are the benefactors of unforeseen technology and years of research which have uncovered treatments to 'sidestep' many of the consequences of getting old, i.e., cataracts, hearing loss, coronary artery disease. It is therefore important to begin the study of the elderly with no prejudices in mind about what to expect with any particular age group. Instead we need to begin to look at individuals who are responding to their environment with fewer strengths and maybe less resilience, rather than as victims of some dreadful process over which they have had no control.

There is a greater number of older people today enjoying the fruits of their labor, having planned successfully for their retirement years and having the good health to find pleasure in their daily lives. Financial analysts give much of the credit for our growing economy to the elderly who have the disposable income to keep travel agents, new car dealers, and home builders in business. It is also not unusual to hear of grandparents who indulge their offspring with generous gifts, educational expenses for their grandchildren and down payment money for homes and cars, providing their families with benefits which could otherwise not be affordable.

The unfortunate truth is that there is a growing number of elderly who have not the resources to enjoy life to the fullest, who feel they have become a burden not only to society, but often to their families who are reaching deep into their pockets to cover housing, medical and other expenses for themselves. Many suffer substantial reductions in income after retirement, with the threat of loss of independent living, changes in health care benefits and fear of spending down their lifetime savings. In addition, there are those overly trusting elders who have been victims of exploitation by those who may appear to be 'do-gooders.' They fall prey into the hands of criminals hoping to benefit financially from what turns out to be the latest scheme. The elderly poor who lose their good health, experience further difficulties as they face rising costs for insurance, medicine, and hospitalization. The term 'fixed income' is a painful reminder for some who no longer have the potential to meet the demands of their continuing existence.

Chronological age needs only to be used as a point in time, rather than as an explanation for good health or lack thereof. We have come to define functional age as that stage in which the individual continues to interface with his environment without extraneous assistance. Understanding functional age allows us to maximize the patient's autonomy without denying independence and dignity. Age alone cannot explain why certain changes take place nor can it prescribe or differentiate our nursing plans of care.

If we are to provide optimal care for the elderly, to see them with their individual characteristics and human needs, then we must expect to find that some of the natural consequences of the aging process are less than desirable. In reality, there is nothing quite as beautiful as one who has experienced a very full life, whose face and hands alone tell a thousand stories of success and failures, joys and sorrows. There are decades of life to explore and understand. Let us waste no further time.

I. Who are the elderly

  A. There is no historical precedent for the aged in our society.

  1. The social, cultural, economical and emotional impact we are experiencing is a unique phenomenon.

  2. We are falling quickly into the unknown depths of an ocean of unexplored issues regarding the aging process and its complications.

  B. The health care industry will be most seriously affected.

  1. With age comes losses including health, independence, functional and cognitive decline as well as accessibility to and availability of resources.

  2. Holistic medicine encompasses the psychosocial and biologic changes that occur allowing for a comprehensive assessment to be done on the aged client.

  C. The effects of aging have only recently been the subject of extensive research.

  1. What constitutes 'optimal health' for the elderly?

  2. Are the needs of the client taken into consideration when scientific knowledge is applied?

  3. How can we promote and maintain optimal health at each phase of the aging spectrum?

II. The statistics

  A. Life expectancy.

  1. In 1992 . . . There were 18.5 million people in the 65-74 age group. This is eight times more than in 1900.

  2. There were 10.6 million in the 75-84 age group. This is 14 times more than in 1900.

  3. There were 3.3 million in the 85+ age group. This is 26 times more than in 1900.

  B. Rapid growth rate of the older American population.

  1. The estimated population of persons 65 yrs. or older numbered 32.4 million in 1992.

The Outline Series: Geriatric Nursing -- 5

2. There are now 36,000 centenarians in this country.

3. It is predicted that there will be more than 250,000 people reach their 100th birthday by the year 2020.

4. Approximately 1 out of every 8 Americans is over the age of 65, or one out of every 5 households (see figure 1).

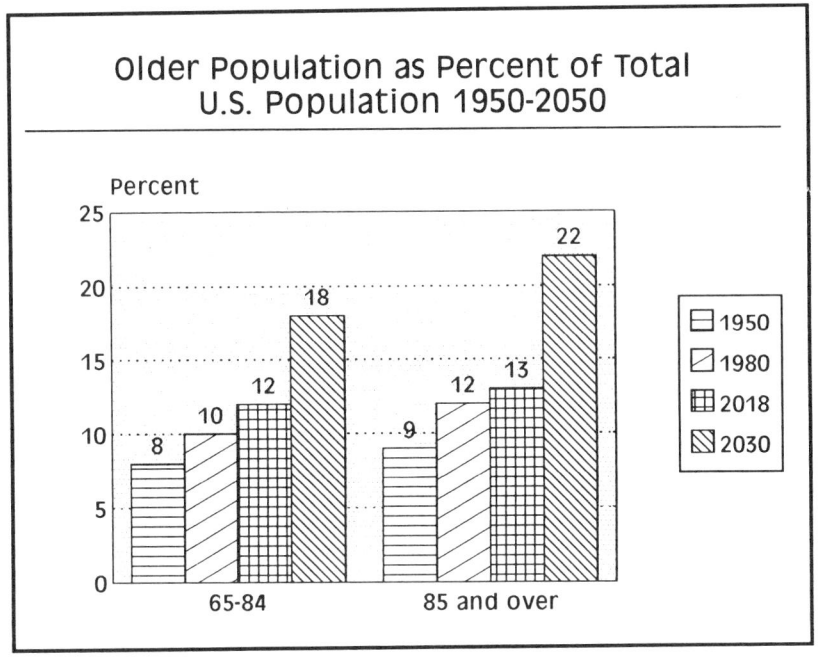

Older Population as Percent of Total U.S. Population 1950-2050

Age group	1950	1980	2018	2030
65-84	8	10	12	18
85 and over	9	12	13	22

Figure 1

5. Approximately 1 of 5 voters is over the age of 65.

6. Half the viewers of prime time television are over the age of 65.

7. Older men reaching the age of 65 in 1991 had an additional 15 yr life expectancy.

8. Older women reaching the age of 65 in 1991 had an additional 17.4 yr life expectancy.

9. In 1992, 2.1 million persons celebrated their 65th birthday; 5700/day -- 1.6 million persons age 65 died, resulting in a net increase of 1420 persons/day.

10. In the year 2030, there will be 70 million older adults, or more than twice the number that were alive in 1990. The implications for the health care industry are inconceivable.

C. Future Predictions/'Baby Boomers' in the next century

1. By the year 2050, 25% of the population will be over the age of 65.

2. The needs for extensive, comprehensive health care will be imperative, just to maintain current levels of functioning.

3. As disability occurs, the number of caregivers and services must multiply to meet the needs.

4. Combined effects of 'ZPG' (Zero Population Growth) of the '70's, along with increasing longevity, has resulted in fewer persons of working age relative to the older population.

5. The 'Dependency Ratio' will dictate the delivery of care in the next decade.

6. In China, with mandated one-child families, a single individual will be responsible for two aging parents.

III. Chronologic, functional age and educational background

A. Differentiation in terminology dictates plan of care

1. Dates on the calendar denote only the passing of time, not the level of physical activity, or decline, nor the response to it.

2. Daily efforts to stay physically and mentally 'spry' yield the greatest dividends.

B. Aging effects are individualized, based on genetic factors, environment health habits and heritage.

1. The octogenarians of the 1990's are a unique segment of the population.

2. These seniors were entering the world at the turn of the century, the days of the literal horse and buggy.

3. They were born long before births routinely took place in hospitals, before the invention of the 'flying machine', and the television.

4. There was no air-conditioning, indoor plumbing, or microwaves.

5. There had been two world wars, the tragedies of the Titanic and the Hindenburg, the atrocities of Auschwitz and the epidemics which killed their infant brothers and sisters.

6. It was not uncommon for children to die from diphtheria, measles and pneumonia without the supplements of formula and multivitamins.

7. The majority of today's elders, were raised in rural areas, where women tended to the home, the children and their older relatives who usually all lived under one roof.

8. Life expectancy in the 1900's was approximately 50 yrs. of age, leaving young wives widowed, raising children alone.

9. The oldest son was first to take over as 'man of the house,' forsaking educational pursuits to help his widowed mother.

10. Young women were often married by the age of 18, beginning their families of 6 or more children very early in life.

11. It was not unusual for extended families to live with their relatives, increasing the responsibilities and expenses for the head of household.

C. Educational differences

Educational standards have changed dramatically in this century. Society has evolved from the one-room school house, to highly specialized forums for teaching today's youth. Historically, children were taught the 'Three R's', (reading, writing, and 'rithmetic) in preparation for the real world. If there were needs at home or in the family business, education was forsaken. For many, elementary school was the highest level of education available.

1. The 'over 80' age group is the least educated segment in our society

2. Approximately 50% have graduated from high school

3. Approximately 10% have a college education

4. Lack of formal education plays a prohibitive role in later life career choices

As for high school, there were few who ever achieved 'Senior' status. Our grandparents grew up during a time when learning father's trade was the only choice for most young men. Women were taught the domestic skills necessary to maintain home and family. Advanced education was something not available nor needed by most. Those that were considered to be 'high achievers' struggled to obtain college degrees during World War I, a depression and a rapidly changing economic climate.

D. Year of school completed for males and females 65 yrs of age and over:

	Males	Females
8 years or less	24%	28%
12 years	47%	44%
16 years	9%	16%

(Statistical Abstract of the U.S.)

E. Ethnic differences

The percent of elderly today who have completed high school:

- Blacks 33%
- Hispanics 26%
- Caucasians . . . 63%

IV. The Labor Force

A. Economic Issues

1. Recent economic slumps have forced elders out of their careers prematurely.

2. Retirement benefits and income potential are lost.

3. Financial needs may dictate continued employment for some.

4. Investments and other supplemental income may allow the choice to retire.
B. Retirement
   1. No longer mandated at age 65
   2. Insufficient funds and inadequate planning on the part of the employer may lead to down-sizing at the expense of the older worker.
   3. The Equal Employment Opportunity Commission (EEOC) and the U.S. Commission on Civil Rights handle discrimination cases against workers who have been mistreated in the work place.
   4. By age 64, more than 45% of this age group have left the labor force.
   5. By age 70 only 10 % of men and 0.3% of women remain in the work force.
   6. Those that remain in the work force after age 70 are doing service or clerical work.
   7. Partial retirement is not uncommon, with partial responsibilities and flexible hours enabling the older adult to remain employed.
   8. Labor force participation by women since 1950 has nearly doubled, changing role expectations for older females.
   9. Older workers are increasingly joining 'temp teams' after retiring from full time work.
   10. Senior recruits within the temp agency are found to be valuable employees with professional skills and excellent training.
C. Life after retirement
   1. Today's retirees are actively involved in politics, educational pursuits, volunteer activities and travel.
   2. Octogenarians and beyond have remained politically, in the entertainment world, and as consultants in various fields.

3. Offering financial support to children and grandchildren is an option for many, providing money for education, housing, vacations and unpaid bills.

4. Recent studies indicate that nearly 2 million grandparents are raising their children's offspring without the parent in the home.

5. The median income for grandparents raising children is $18,000, nearly 1/2 that of the traditional family.

6. Single grandparent caregivers are usually women, 93%

7. Current legislation prohibits grandparents from receiving Aid to Dependent Families, covering the grandchildren on health insurance policies and being entitled to foster care reimbursement.

VI. Levels of Income

A. Decreased income

1. Income for the elderly usually drops by approximately 33% after retirement

2. 20% of those over the age of 85 and over are at the poverty level.

B. Income estimates

1. For older males is approximately $15,000.

2. For older females is approximately $8,000. (1992)

3. Median income for homes where the head of household is over the age of 65 (see figure 2):
   - Caucasian $25,000
   - Black $16,600
   - Hispanics $19,200

4. Poverty levels across ethnic boundaries
   - Caucasian 33%
   - Black 22%
   - Hispanic 11%

The Outline Series: Geriatric Nursing -- 11

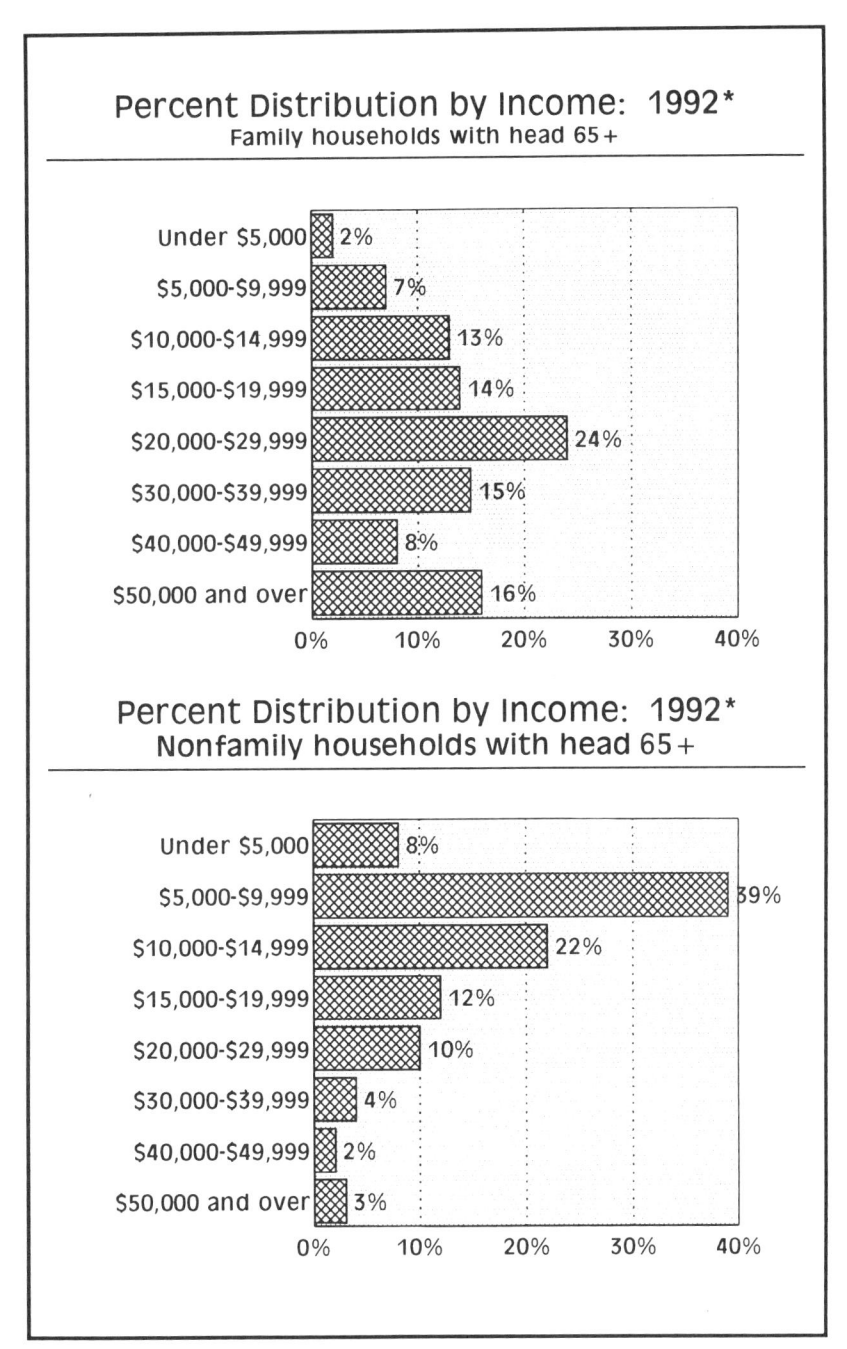

Percent Distribution by Income: 1992*
Family households with head 65+

Income	Percent
Under $5,000	2%
$5,000-$9,999	7%
$10,000-$14,999	13%
$15,000-$19,999	14%
$20,000-$29,999	24%
$30,000-$39,999	15%
$40,000-$49,999	8%
$50,000 and over	16%

Percent Distribution by Income: 1992*
Nonfamily households with head 65+

Income	Percent
Under $5,000	8%
$5,000-$9,999	39%
$10,000-$14,999	22%
$15,000-$19,999	12%
$20,000-$29,999	10%
$30,000-$39,999	4%
$40,000-$49,999	2%
$50,000 and over	3%

Figure 2

5. Poverty rates for women are greater than men - 15% to 8%.
6. Income for the elderly may come from varied sources
   - Social Security benefits;
   - Pensions;
   - Wages;
   - Dividends from investments;
   - Depletion of savings accounts.
7. For 40% of older couples, the major source of income is their Social Security check.

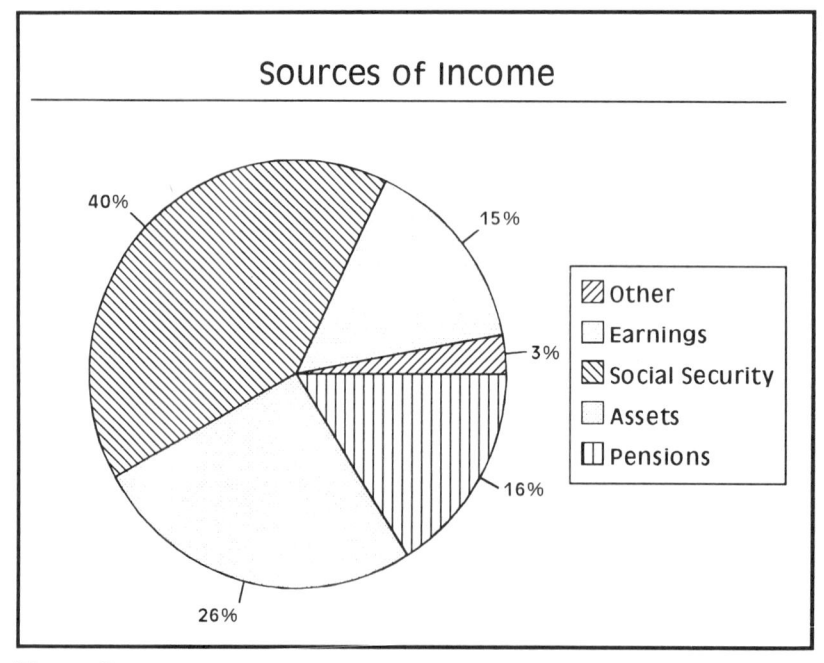

Sources of Income

- 40% Social Security
- 26% Assets
- 16% Pensions
- 15% Earnings
- 3% Other

Figure 3

8. For 26%, the major source of income is from investments.
9. For 16%, the major source of income is from pensions.

C. Cost vs. Income
   1. The average Social Security check today is approximately $550.00.

2. The average cost for health care per year for persons over the age of 65 is $5,000.00.

3. 25% of health care costs are assumed by the individual; 75% of health care costs are assumed by Medicare, Medicaid and private coverage.

4. Over 4 million elderly people are living at the poverty level today, with average incomes of less than $8500.

VII. Housing

A. Where the elderly live

1. Approximately 75% of the elderly own their homes and 75% of these are mortgage free.

2. Studies show that a great majority of these homes are first and only dwellings, often with sub-standard insulation, sub-obtimal energy efficiency and are structurally inadequate.

3. More than 65% of these homes were built prior to 1950.

4. There is often little discretionary income directed toward remodeling and repairs.

5. Older single women living alone outnumber men 2:1.

6. Internationally, those over the age of 65 living alone;
   - Sweden 40%
   - Netherlands 32%
   - Germany 39%
   - France 33%
   - United Kingdom 30%
   - United States 30%
   - Canada 20%
   - Japan 9%

B. Housing alternatives

As capacity and functional abilities deteriorate, older persons are more likely to leave their independent style of living, whether voluntarily or not to join extended family, or choose from a variety of senior living arrangements, offering various degrees of supervision and assistance. Statistically, the greater the age, the more likely is placement in a skilled nursing facility. (See figure 4 on pages 15 & 16.)

1. Congregate residences

2. ECHO (Elderly Cottage Housing Options)

3. Senior retirement centers

4. Assisted living centers

5. Nursing homes

Once activities of daily living (ADL's) are no longer an independent function, 24 hour supervision and assistance may be required, leading individuals and families to consider long-term care placement. Only 5% of the elderly reside in long-term care facilities, due to illness and disability rather than abandonment by family. (See figures 5 17,18, and 19.)

The Outline Series: Geriatric Nursing -- 15

Figure 4, page 1 of 2
Percent of Persons 65 Years of Age and Over Who Reported Receiving the Help of another Person with Performing Activities of Daily Living, by Race, Sex, and Age: United States

(Data are based on household interviews of the civilian noninstitutionalized population.)

Race, sex and age	Total	Eating	Toileting	Dressing	Bathing	Transferring[1]	Walking	Getting Outside
	Number of persons in thousands			Percent				
Race								
White	24,753	1.1	2.3	4.2	5.6	3.0	4.5	6.1
All other	2,784	*0.6	3.5	6.1	9.4	5.2	5.8	7.8
Sex								
Male	11,357	1.0	1.9	3.9	4.3	2.6	3.1	3.8
Female	16,181	1.1'	2.8	4.7	7.2	3.7	5.8	8.0
Age								
65-74 years	16,987	0.8	1.4	2.9	3.2	2.1	2.6	3.2
75-84 years	8,552	1.1	3.3	5.4	8.6	4.0	6.4	9.2
65 years and over	27,538	1.1	2.4	4.4	6.0	3.2	4.6	6.3
75 years and over	10,551	1.6	4.1	6.8	10.6	5.0	8.0	11.3
85 years and over	1,999	4.1	7.5	12.6	19.0	9.4	14.8	20.6

Figure 4, page 2 of 2

Race, sex and age	Total Number of persons in thousands	Eating	Toileting	Dressing	Bathing	Trans-ferring[1]	Walking	Getting Outside
				Percent				
Male								
65-74 years	7,490	0.9	1.5	3.2	3.3	2.3	2.3	2.7
75-84 years	3,251	*0.6	1.9	4.2	4.9	2.3	3.7	4.8
65 years and over	11,357	1.0	1.9	3.9	4.3	2.6	3.1	3.8
75 years and over	3,866	1.3	2.5	5.2	6.4	3.2	4.5	6.0
85 years and over	615	*4.7	*5.9	10.0	14.1	7.8	8.3	12.8
Female								
65-74 years	9,496	0.6	1.3	2.6	3.1	2.0	2.8	3.5
75-84 years	5,301	1.3	4.1	6.1	10.9	5.0	8.0	11.9
65 years and over	16,181	1.1	2.8	4.7	7.2	3.7	5.8	8.0
75 years and over	6,685	1.8	5.0	7.7	13.0	6.1	10.0	14.4
85 years and over	1,384	*3.9	8.3	13.8	21.2	10.1	17.8	24.1

[1]Transferring means getting in and out of a bed or chair.
*Figure does not meet standards of reliability.
NOTE: Persons reported as not performing an activity of daily living (ADL) were classified with those reported as receiving help with that ADL.
Source: National Center for Health Statistics; data from the National Health Interview Survey 1986 Functional Limitations Supplement.

Figure 5 page 1 of 2 -- Nursing and Related Care Facilities, by Selected Characteristics: 1991

(Excludes hospital-based nursing homes which numbered 767 with 51,897 residents in 1991. Based on the National Health Provider Inventor.)

CHARACTERISTIC	TOTAL FACILITIES				NURSING HOMES[1]				BOARD & CARE HOMES[1]			
	Homes	Beds (1000)	Avg. no. of beds	Occu-pancy rate	Homes	Beds (1000)	Avg. no. of beds	Occu-pancy rate	Homes	Beds (1000)	Avg. no. of beds	Occu-pancy rate
Total	33,006	1,921	58	90.0	14,744	1,559	106	91.5	18,262	362	20	83.6
Region												
Northeast	5,834	414	71	93.5	2,654	328	124	95.3	3,180	86	27	86.6
Midwest	9,142	583	64	89.7	5,137	519	101	90.3	4,005	64	16	84.7
South	9,499	609	64	89.6	4,708	504	107	90.9	4,791	106	22	83.0
West	8,531	315	37	86.8	2,245	209	93	89.6	6,286	106	17	81.3
Ownership												
Government	1,570	113	72	92.3	725	100	138	93.5	845	13	16	83.8
Proprietary	24,256	1,349	56	89.0	10,522	1,087	103	90.6	13,734	262	19	82.6
Nonprofit	7,180	459	64	92.2	3,497	372	106	93.5	3,683	87	24	86.8

Figure 5, page 2 of 2 -- Nursing and Related Care Facilities, by Selected Characteristics: 1991

CHARACTERISTIC	TOTAL FACILITIES				NURSING HOMES[1]				BOARD & CARE HOMES[1]			
	Homes	Beds (1000)	Avg. no. of beds	Occu-pancy rate	Homes	Beds (1000)	Avg. no. of beds	Occu-pancy rate	Homes	Beds (1000)	Avg. no. of beds	Occu-pancy rate
Size												
Fewer than 10 beds	10,025	53	5	83.9	165	1	5	81.6	9,860	52	5	83.9
10 to 24 beds	5,281	82	15	85.5	398	7	18	88.5	4,883	74	15	85.2
25 to 49 beds	3,381	124	37	87.9	1,590	61	39	91.1	1,791	62	35	84.9
50 to 74 beds	3,792	229	60	90.9	3,050	184	60	92.1	742	44	60	85.8
75 to 99 beds	2,795	245	88	90.2	2,401	211	88	91.2	394	34	86	83.8
100 to 199 beds	6,497	854	132	90.8	6,028	792	131	91.5	469	62	132	81.9
200 to 299 beds	941	217	231	90.1	846	196	231	91.4	95	22	228	79.0
300 to 499 beds	248	89	358	89.5	224	80	359	91.0	24	8	347	75.5
500 beds or more	46	29	633	90.8	42	26	625	92.1	4	3	721	78.8

[1] These facilities hzve three or more beds.
[2] These facilities offer no nursing services and provide only personal care or superviwsor care. Excludes board and care homes for the metnally retarded.

Source: U.S. National Center for Health Statistics, *Advance Data From Vital and Health Statistics*, No. 244; and unpublished data.

VIII. Marital and family status

A. Men/Women/Couples

1. Older men are more likely to be married (80%) than older women (52%)

2. In the over 75 age group, women are more likely to be widowed than men (66% - 24%) (see figure 6).

3. Older women, once widowed, receive the bulk of their care from their adult children, primarily the daughter or daughter-in-law. (see figure 7)

4. Married older couples who live in comfortable surroundings seem to be able to cope more effectively with life's changes and losses than those elderly living alone.

5. In 1990, almost 75,000 persons over the age of 65 got married, most of them for the second time.

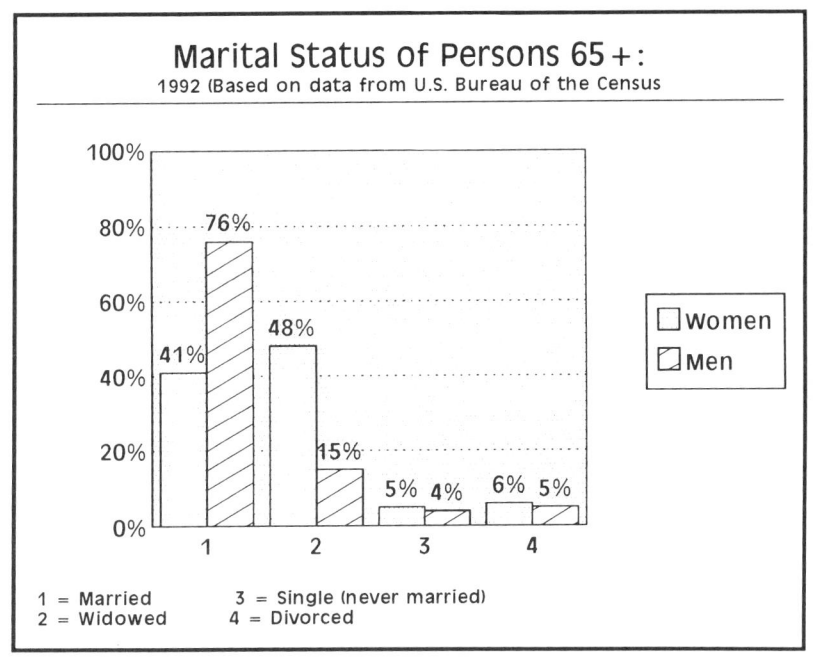

Marital Status of Persons 65+:
1992 (Based on data from U.S. Bureau of the Census)

Category	Women	Men
1 = Married	41%	76%
2 = Widowed	48%	15%
3 = Single (never married)	5%	4%
4 = Divorced	6%	5%

Figure 6

20 -- *Where Are The Elderly*

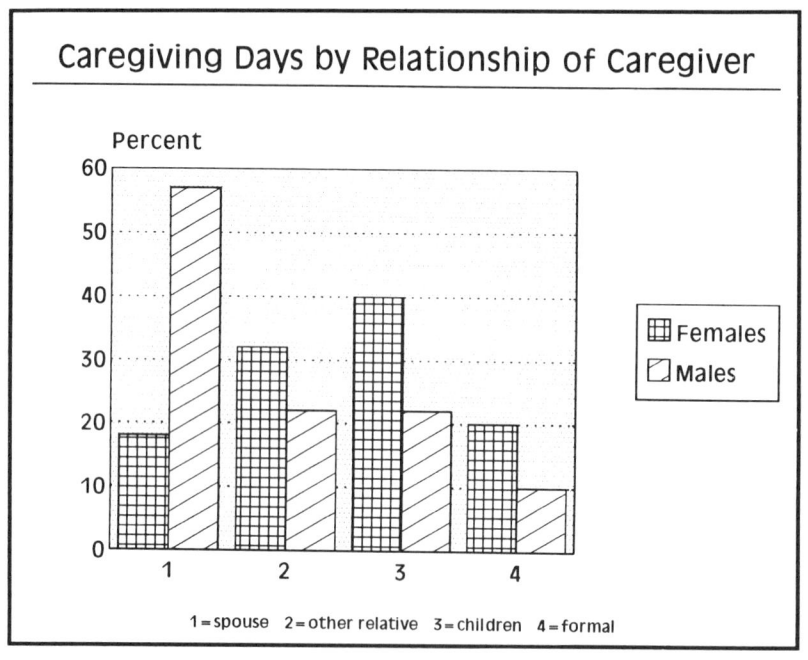

Caregiving Days by Relationship of Caregiver

Percent

Females
Males

1 = spouse 2 = other relative 3 = children 4 = formal

Figure 7

    6. When an older, married individual becomes disabled, the spouse is the most likely caregiver. When the spouse is absent or unable, the adult children are most likely to provide the necessary care.

    7. Older couples tend to pay more attention to personal hygiene, daily routine, nutrition and home maintenance than single older people.

B. Family Status

    1. While the majority of the elderly live with their spouse, a large percentage live alone or with other relatives.

    2. Relatives are the primary source for assistance when health and physical functioning begin to deteriorate.

    3. The female adult-child caregiver is career-oriented (55%) and therefore must reconcile the demands of family, job stressors, and parental care.

    (See figure 8.)

The Outline Series: Geriatric Nursing -- 21

Living Arrangements of Persons 65+: 1992

PERCENTS

- Men: 1=74, 2=19, 3=7
- Women: 1=40, 2=42, 3=18

1 = Living with spouse
2 = Living with other relatives
3 = Living alone or with non-relatives

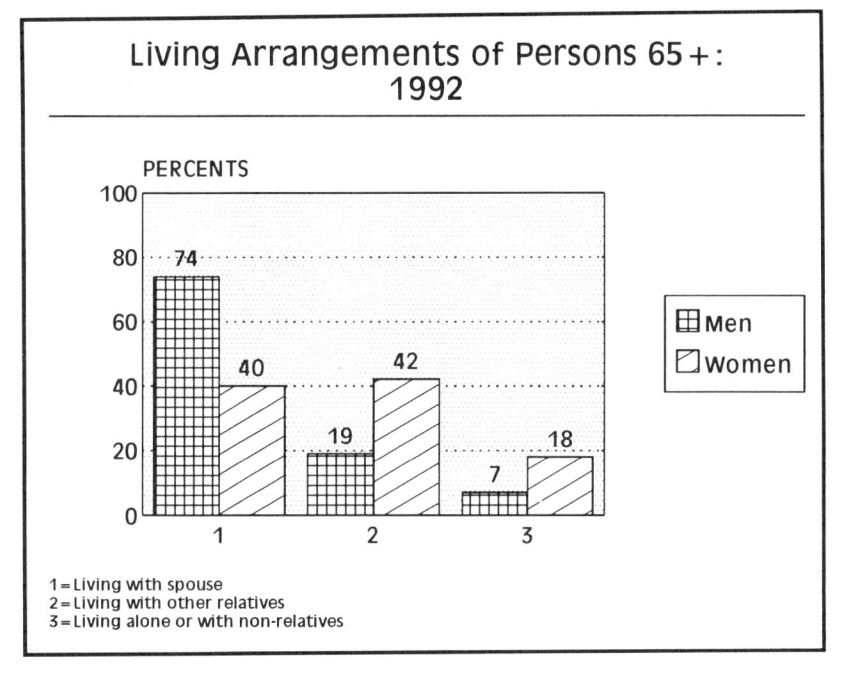

Figure 8

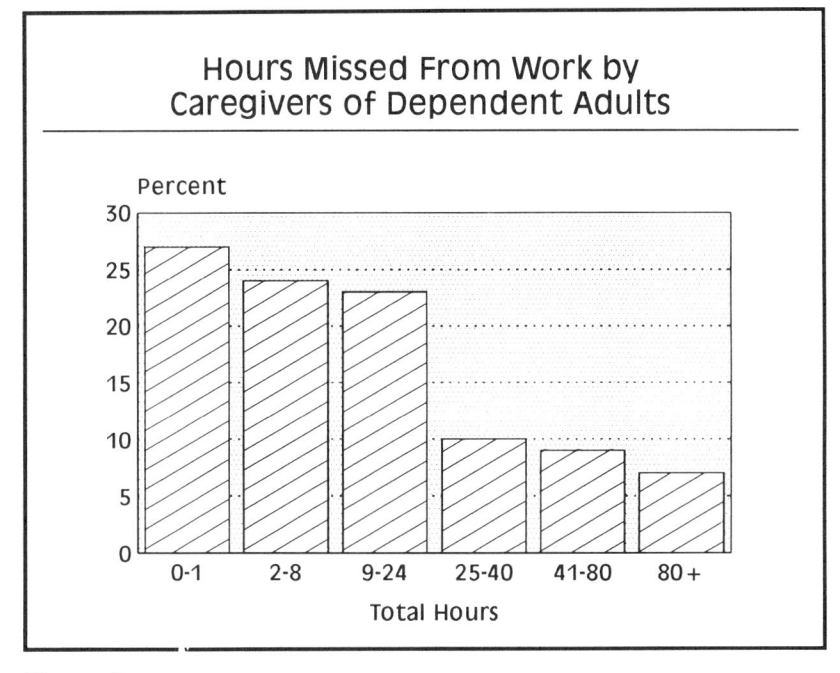

Hours Missed From Work by Caregivers of Dependent Adults

Percent by Total Hours:
- 0-1: ~27
- 2-8: ~24
- 9-24: ~23
- 25-40: ~10
- 41-80: ~9
- 80+: ~7

Figure 9

IX. Ageism

For many years, the elderly were looked upon as a group of individuals who had lost their ability to work, live independently, think coherently and remain a productive part of society. Not only are these and many other perceptions wrong, they constitute a theory described by Robert Butler in 1969 as "Ageism."

A. Misconceptions

1. The youthful society in which we live perceives those who are not productive and technologically proficient as somehow less than equal and less deserving of the bounty of resources available today.

2. Historically, other subgroups of the population, such as the handicapped or underprivileged have also experienced this type of national prejudice.

3. Misinformation about the elderly leads to biases and discriminatory treatment, based on age, disability or residential status, i.e. a nursing home.

B. Discrimination

1. Recent studies conducted at the National Institute on Aging have concluded that the elderly do not receive the same treatment nor options when seeking medical attention.

2. A study of 250 cardiac patients over the age of 60 received significantly less information than their younger counterparts regarding resources, health manage-ment, and health promotion.

3. The National Institute on Aging conducted a study which revealed almost 50% of those physicians queried believed that the elderly should not receive maximum evaluation for acute illness.

4. Though old age is not always a preferred state, alternatives for maximizing health as one experiences the aging process are numerous. Choices for and about health care should be given to the client without regard to age or cognitive ability.

The Outline Series: Geriatric Nursing -- 23

X. Health Status

A. Chronicity

1. Approximately 30% of those over the age of 65 have negative perceptions about their physical health, due to a gradual decline in physical abilities, effects of diminished functioning of vital organs, i.e. cardiac output and tidal volume capacity as well as less than optimal return to baseline after an acute episode.

2. Chronic illness is common among the elderly, work-related activities.

   - Older workers average 34 days per year of restricted activity at work due to illness or injury.
   - Approximately 1/2 of those reported sick days are spent in bed.

3. Chronic conditions which most often affect the elderly:

   a. Arthritis 53%
   b. Hypertension 43%
   c. Hearing impairment 52%
   d. Heart disease 40%
   e. Orthopedic problems 18%
   f. Cataracts 22%
   g. Sinusitis 14%
   h. Diabetes 9%
   i. Tinnitus 9%
   j. Varicosities 8%

B. Hospitalization

1. The elderly are responsible for 35% of all hospital stays.

   - The average length of stay in the hospital is 8.6 days for older people, compared to only 5.2 days for the younger adult.

2. The number of hospital stays for the elderly has decreased 5.6 days since 1968 and 2.1 further days since 1980.

   - The trend for early discharge has had a monumental effect on the home health care industry.

3. The elderly spend approximately 40% of their health care budget for costs related to hospitalization;
   - 20% for physician services
   - 20% for nursing home care
4. Benefits from Medicare and Medicaid ($72 billion and $20 billion, respectively) accounted for two-thirds of health expenditures for the elderly, as opposed to 20% spent for persons younger than 65.

C. Functional ability despite chronicity

Factors which predict a high level of functioning;

- High family income
- Absence of hypertension
- Absence of arthritis and back pain
- Absence of smoking
- Normal body weight
- Moderate or no alcohol consumption
- Continued physical ability
- Lack of cardiovascular disease
- High level of education

XII. The elderly female

A. Statistically
1. In 1992, there were 19.2 million older women, compared to 13.0 million men.
2. The ratio of women to men in long term care facilities is 10:1.
3. Since women typically outlive men, they experience a unique number of disease processes in their later years, creating a new demand for health care services.

B. Health care needs

1. The need for appropriate health promotional materials as well as screening tools is imperative in today's aging population of women.

2. Medical research which explores the differences in healthy aging among women has just begun, leaving vast amounts of data to be explored.

3. Women have more episodes of illness than men, with less likelihood of mortality, with a resultant increase in their period of morbidity.

C. Chronic conditions

1. Many of the chronic conditions which have plagued older women for decades, are now being seen in men who are extending the life expectancy every year. Ironically, the conditions which older women have tolerated stoically, seemingly are rendering men incapable of carrying out major activities. (28% men to 8% women)

2. Conditions which are most often seen in older women;

    a. Arthritis 50%

    b. Hypertension 40%

    c. Hearing impairment 30%

    d. Visual impairment 10%

    e. Women also have more frequent diagnoses of osteoporosis, nutritional disorders, depression and cancer. "In older women, health status cannot be adequately assessed nor can primary and secondary preventive care be provided by merely performing periodic screening."

C. Health promotion

1. A multi-disciplinary approach which involves a thorough assessment of physical and mental health, and an evaluation of basic and social functioning is the best approach.

2. It is essential to understand the implications brought about by any impairment in order to develop appropriate plans of care.

3. Prevention of disease and promotion of strengths is the most effective means for treating the older female.

XIII. Routine health maintenance for older women

A. The physical exam should include not only the height, weight, and baseline vital signs, but also a thorough physical and social history. In addition, risk factors based on physical, functional and cognitve limitations need to be addressed.

1. A gynecologic exam, including breast exam and pap smear should be included to rule out abnormalities, lesions and possible dynsfunction.

2. It is a misconception that women who are past their childbearing years no longer need gynecologic exams. (See figure 10)

B. There are many changes that occur in older women in later years:

1. Atrophic changes in the vulva and vagina,

2. Pelvic relaxation with uterine prolapse and stress incontinence,

3. Hormonal changes including breast atrophy, evidence of facial hair, and loss of bone density due to decreased estrogen production.

C. 36% of new breast cancers and 42% of deaths caused by breast carcinomas occur in women 65 years and older.

1. Statistically, the prognosis is the same despite the older age, yet the increased mortality reflects either delayed diagnosis or a less aggressive treatment modality.

2. Because the breasts of older women are pendulous or atrophic, nodules or lumps may not be easily detected.

XIV. Nutrition

A. A thorough nutritional assessment is also an important part of the physical exam.

1. 30% of women between the ages of 65 and 74 are obese.

Recommended frequency of various components of periodic history taking and examination in healthy older women

COMPONENT	FREQUENCY
Questioning regarding:	
Diet	
Physical activity	Annually from age 65
Tobacco, alcohol, or drug abuse Functional status at home	
Caregiving tasks	
Immunizations	
Tetanus and diphtheria booster	Every 10 yr
Influenza vaccine	Annually
Pneumococcal vaccine	Once
Physical examination	
Height and weight	Annually
Blood pressure	Annually
Visual acuity	Physician's discretion
Hearing	Physician's discretion
Clinical breast examination	Annually
Laboratory procedures	
Nonfasting total blood cholesterol	Every 4 yr after age 60
Fasting plasma glucose	Physician's discretion
Dipstick urinalysis or urine culture	Physician's discretion
Mammogram	Annually after age 50
Tuberculin PPD skin test	When entering communal living arrangements
Pap smear	Every 1 to 3 yr
Fecal occult blood testing or sigmoidoscopy	Annually

2. Diet may be the key to preventing many medical problems affecting this segment, such as stroke, disease, orthopedic difficulties and constipation.
   B. Evaluation of weight in relation to normal body weight for age is essential.
      1. Loss of significant weight is a greater problem for these individuals than obesity, which affects more younger women.
      2. Significant weight loss is defined as more than 1% - 2% of body weight per week.
   C. Weight loss in older women may be due to poor dentition, depression, malignant disease, or socioeconomic factors.

XV. Osteoporosis

   A. Osteoporosis primarily affects postmenopausal women, usually around age 50.
      1. More than 90% of the 20 million Americans with osteoporosis are women.
      2. Statistically, 25% of these women will suffer bone fractures because of decreased bone mass.
      3. There are more than 250,000 hip fractures per year with a high morbidity and approximately 15% mortality.
   B. There are two types of osteoporosis; primary and secondary
      1. Primary osteoporosis occurs shortly after the onset of menopause and may be partially responsible for the high incidence of hip and wrist fractures.
      2. Secondary osteoporosis occurs mostly after the age of 75 and is slightly less prevalent in women than men. It is usually excessive use of alcohol and tobacco, hormone deficiencies and chronic illness.
   C. Recent studies have shown that estrogen supplements during the early stages of menopause can slow the loss of bone mass.
      1. Continued use of estrogen has been indicated as beneficial in prevention of heart disease and some dementias.

2. Despite the benefits of ERT (estrogen replacement therapy) the inconvenience of continuing menstrual cycles may be unattractive

D. The National Institute of Health Consensus Development Conference on Osteoporosis makes the following recommendations;

1. Estrogen supplementation beginning at the early stages of menopause

2. Calcium supplementation should be started approximately 10 years before menopause in daily doses of 1000 mg/day.

3. Weight bearing exercises, such as walking, dancing, regularly.

E. Problematic habits which increase the risk of losing bone mass include;

1. Lack of regular weight-bearing exercise

2. Inadequate intake of calcium

3. High intake of fiber (which interferes with the absorption of calcium)

4. Smoking and alcohol

5. Daily intake of products with caffeine

XVI. Mental health

Dysfunction in the area of mental health for the elderly may stem from social difficulties, such as multiple losses, financial decline, loneliness and isolation. Those that do seek help, usually do so with the great encouragement of family, friends and religious support.

A. Differences in feelings of health

1. Women generally seek medical attention more often than their male counterparts.

2. It is also suggested that women are more sensitive to changes in physical and mental health, therefore responding to feelings of poor health promptly.

3. Men have historically been socialized to deny the need for medical attention, wanting to appear stoic and somewhat invincible.

B. Mental health in women historiclly changes over time

1. Women of the 1930's, reaching menopause and often simultaneously 'empty nest syndrome,' experienced severe psychologic and emotional impairment.

2. Mental hospitals, as they were called, were filled with middle-aged women diagnosed with 'involutional melancholia.'

3. Changes in women's roles in the last 25 years, has brought about a drastic reduction in the number of women with symptoms who need hospitalization.

4. Women suffering impaired mental function over the age of 40 has decreased by 50%.

5. Careers and challenging mid-life opportunities have brought about a resurgence and renewed sense of purpose as women move into the second fifty years of their lives.

C. Availability of mental health services

1. Current trends have improved the recognition and development of gero-psychiatric services.

2. Physicians, elder clinics and community organizations are excellent sources of referral for those in need of mental health evaluations.

SUMMARY

Growing old has taken on an entirely new meaning for the 'Silver Generation.' This group has become not only a powerful component in the economic and political world, but also the subject of thousands of publications addressing needs, challenges and discoveries for today's society. The elderly constitute a diverse and fascinating component in every community in which they reside. Their history is not only unique, but one from which we can develop a better understanding of their individualized perceptions and requirements of the health care team. All humans require social interaction, a sense of purpose and treatment with respect and dignity. As age begins to effect the individual's ability to maintain self, the demands for quality support increased proportionately. Health professionals must respond to these needs creatively and with empathy. Though it is recognized that life inevitably must come to an end, the plea for the highest quality of care never ceases.

References

1990 Census of Population and Housing. U.S. Department of Commerce

Department of Health and Human Services "Hours Missed From Work"

Ebersole and Hess. *Toward Healthy Aging* Mosby, Inc. 1994

Friedan, Betty. *Fountain of Age,* Simon and Schuster

Schick, Renee. *Statistical Handbook on Aging Americans*. Onyx Press, 1994

South-Paul, Jeannette, and Cheryl Woodson, MD. "Optimal Care of Older Women", Vol 91: #4, 3/92

Stone, Robin, Calferata. "Caregivers of the Frail Elderly: A National Profile" The Gerontologist vol 27 no. 5

U.S. Census Bureau 1990. "Assets, Pensions, etc."

U.S. Census Bureau 1990. "Marital Status"

U.S. Census Bureau 1990. "Nursing Home Populations by Region, Division and State"

U.S. Census Bureau 1990. "Older Population as Percent of Total Population"

U.S. Census Bureau 1990. "Percent Distribution by Income"

U.S. Census Bureau. "Living Arrangements of Person 65"

U.S. Department of Health and Human Services. "Percent Having Difficulty and Receiving Help"

U.S. Preventive Services Task Force. *Recommended Frequency of Various Components of Health History.* Post Graduate Medicine, vol. 91., no. 4., March 1992

Vierck, Elizabeth. *Fact Book on Aging*, ABC-CLIO Inc.

Wolff, Michael. *Where We Stand: Can America Make It In the Global Race for Wealth, Health and Happiness*

Unit 1 - Chapter 2

Who Are the Elderly

Though we are often able to generalize about the similarities in the elderly population, we must keep in mind their uniqueness and individuality. There are as many differences in functional, cognitive and emotional qualities among the aged as there are stars in the heavens. There as as many differences as grains of sand. Focusing on strengths instead of weaknesses, looking at history instead of textbook parameters and listening to the real issues that are brought to our attention creates a customized perspective and unbiased knowledge base about this fascinating 'silver segment.'

As we continue to explore the characteristics of this special group, we will also look at the geographics of the older American and the effect of transition as the individuals begins to lose independent functioning.

I. The price of aging in the '90's.

    A. Each year of successful living brings about a series of challenges for the older adult, the caregiver and those who must provide services for this everchanging segment.

        1. Today's modern miracles of advanced medications, technology and procedures, paradoxically not only extended life for the elderly client, but also the related moral, ethical and financial dilemmas.

        2. By-pass grafting, pacemakers and a sophisticated blend of vasodilators, ionotropics and diuretics have provided a much healthier lifestyle for millions.

        3. The cost is most than $160 billion dollars per year to this country; and for some, approximately one-third of their health care allottment is spent during the last two weeks of life.

    B. Where are the elderly?

        1. More than 90% of the elderly population are living in the community; shopping, driving, vacationing, attending the theater, and contributing in a variety of ways to the economy.

- These elders can be described as healthy, energetic, optimistic and resourceful, living life to the fullest.
    2. Greater numbers are now attending classes, pursuing second and third careers, serving as consultants and volunteering in thousands of organizations.
    3. They are donating their time to religious and political causes, philanthropic and social orders, such as the ELKS, the Shriners and the Knights of Columbus.
    4. There is an increasing number of elders caring for a disabled spouse, raising grandchildren, and providing respite for members of their own or church families.
C. Georgraphic characteristics
    1. California has more 85 yr. olds in residence than any other state in the nation; 285,000.
    2. Alaska has the fewest number of elderly; 22,000.
    3. New York City claims more than 1 million individuals over the age of 65
    4. More than 20% of the population in Florida are over the 65 year mark - The majority of these residents have moved in from the colder Northeast and Midwest regions. (see diagram 1 on following pages)
    5. More than one third of older persons in the United States live in the southern part of the country.
    6. Less than one fifth of the elderly live in the Western states, with the remainder, excluding the South in the Midwest and Northeast.
    7. Elders who move to the Sunbelt are generally more affluent, and therfore benefit, rather than handicap the new environment.
    8. The amount of money Florida will have gained from persons over age 60 who have retired there from 1985 to 1990 was over $6 billion.
    9. The elderly left behind in the Snowbelt tend to be older and have fewer financial resources.

Rank Order of States, by Selected Characteristics of the 65+ Population: 1989

Number of People 65+

Rank*	State	Number (000)s
(x)	U.S., total	30,984
(1)	California	3,071
(2)	New York	2,341
(3)	Florida	2,277
(4)	Pennsylvania	1,819
(5)	Texas	1,714
(6)	Illinois	1,437
(7)	Ohio	1,399
(8)	Michigan	1,100
(9)	New Jersey	1,021
(13)	Massachusetts	813
(10)	North Carolina	798
(15)	Missoursi	719
(14)	Indiana	694

People 65+ as percent of state's population

Rank	State	Percent
(x)	U.S., total	12.5
1	Florida	18.0
2	Pennsylvania	15.1
3	Iowa	15.1
4	Rhode Island	14.8
5	Arkansas	14.8
6	West Virginia	14.6
7	South Dakota	14.4
8	Missouri	13.9
9	Nebraska	13.9
10	Oregon	13.9
11	North Dakota	13.9
12	Massachusets	13.8
13	Kansas	13.7

Percent change in number of peopole 65+, 1980-1989

Rank	State	Percent
(x)	U.S., total	21.3
1	Alaska	88.3
2	Nevada	84.5
3	Hawaii	56.6
4	Arizona	51.1
5	New Mexico	38.5
6	South Carolina	35.9
7	Florida	34.9
8	Delaware	34.3
9	Utah	34.1
10	North Carolina	32.4
11	Washington	31.5
12	Colorado	31.1
13	Virginia	30.0

The Outline Series: Geriatric Nursing -- 35

Rank Order of States, by Selected Characteristics of the 65+ Population: 1989

Number of People 65+				People 65+ as percent of state's population			Percent change in number of people 65+, 1980-1989		
14	(12)	Virginia	657	14	Connecticut	13.6	14	Oregon	29.3
15	(11)	Georgia	653	15	Maine	13.4	15	Idaho	29.3
16	(17)	Wisconsin	652	16	Wisconsin	13.4	16	Maryland	28.6
17	(16)	Tennessee	625	17	Oklahoma	13.3	17	California	27.2
18	(18)	Washington	567	18	New Jersey	13.2	18	Gerogia	26.3
29	(21)	Minnesota	549	19	Montana	13.2	19	Montana	25.4
30	(33)	Arkansas	356	30	Illinois	12.3	30	New Jersey	18.18
31	(32)	Kansas	343	31	North Carolina	12.1	31	Indiana	18.5
32	(31)	Mississippi	326	32	Idaho	11.9	32	Rhode Island	16.5
33	(26)	Colorado	324	3	Washington	11.9	33	Maine	16.2
34	(34)	West Virginia	272	34	Vermont	11.9	34	Vermont	16.1
35	(36)	Nebraska	224	35	Michigan	11.9	35	Wisconsin	15.5
36	(38)	Maine	164	36	Delaware	11.8	38	Kentucky	15.1
37	(37)	New Mexico	161	37	New Hampshire	11.4	37	Minnesota	14.5
38	(43)	Rhode Island	148	38	South Carolina	11.1	38	West Virginia	14.2
39	(35)	Utah	146	39	Louisiana	11.1	39	North Dakota	14.0
40	(42)	New Hampshire	126	40	Nevada	10.9	40	Illinois	13.9

Rank Order of States, by Selected Characteristics of the 65+ Population: 1989

Number of People 65+			People 65+ as percent of state's population			Percent change in number of people 65+, 1980-1989		
41	(40)	Nevada 121	41	Maryland	10.8	41	Oklahoma	13.9
42	(41)	Idaho 121	42	Virginia	10.8	42	Arkansas	13.8
43	(39)	Hawaii 119	43	Hawaii	10.7	43	South Dakota	12.9
44	(44)	Montana 106	44	California	10.6	44	Mississippi	12.7
45	(45)	South Dakota 103	45	New Mexico	10.5	45	Kansas	12.0
46	(47)	North Dakota 92	46	Georgia	10.1	46	Massachusetts	11.9
47	(46)	Delaware 79	47	Texas	10.1	47	Missouri	10.9
48	(48)	Dist of Col. 76	48	Wyoming	9.8	48	Iowa	10.5
49	(49)	Vermont 68	49	Colorado	9.8	49	Nebraska	9.1
50	(51)	Wyoming 46	50	Utah	8.5	50	New York	8.3
51	(50)	Alaska 22	51	Alaska	4.1	51	Dist of Col.	1.8

SOURCE: U.S. Bureau of the Census. "State Population and Household Estimates: July 1, 1989." by Edwin Byerly, *Current Population Reports Series* P-25. No 1058 (March 1990), and unpublished data.

NOTE: All rankings in this table are derived from unrounded numbers and percentages.

* Numbers in parentheses represent rank order of states based on population of all ages in 1989.

(*) Not applicable

The Outline Series: Geriatric Nursing -- 37

10. The state of New York will have lost approximately $3 billions this year from persons over the age of 60 who have chosen to relocate.

11. In their later years, over the age of 80, the elderly tend to leave their retirement communities and move toward family.

12. According to the 1990 census, 74% of the elderly live in metropolitan areas, mostly in suburbs, rather than inner city neighborhoods.

13. Many older Americans choose to stay in their original homes, not just for financial concerns, but also for sentimental reasons. Often the neighborhood changes, leaving them in unsafe, economically deprived surroundings.

14. 25% of the rural community is elderly as opposed to only 12% of the urban areas.

15. More than 90% of the elderly live in the community independently, or with family; approximately 5% live in long-term care facilities.

Countries with MORE than 2 Million Elderly Persons in 1991
(in thousands)

Country	Population aged 65 and over	Country	Population aged 65 and over
China, Mainland	67,967	Bangladesh	3,492
India	32,780	Vietnam	3,196
United States	32,045	Canada	3,140
Japan	15,253	Argentina	3,012
Germany	12,010	Turkey	2,789
United Kingdom	9,025	Nigeria	2,676
Italy	8,665	Romania	2,489
France	8,074	Philippines	2,380
Brazil	6,680	Thailand	2,350
Indonesia	5,962	Yugoslavia	2,328
Spain	5,378	South Korea	2,135
Pakistan	4,734	Egypt	2,077
Poland	3,851	Iran	2,052
Mexico	3,522		

Source: U.S. Bureau of the Census, Kevin Kinsella, Center for International Research, International Data Base

Figure 2

Countries with MORE than 2 Million Elderly Persons in 2020
(in thousands)

Country	Population aged 65 and over
China, Mainland	179,561
India	88,495
United States	53,627
Japan	33,421
Indonesia	22,183
Brazil	18,800
Germany	18,396
Italy	13,078
France	12,119
United Kingdom	12,108
Mexico	10,857
Pakistan	9,678
Nigeria	9,152
Bangladesh	9,057
Spain	8,162
Turkey	7,990
Thailand	7,828
Poland	7,243
Vietnam	6,707
Philippines	6,646
South Korea	6,550
Canada	6,404
Egypt	5,680
Iran	5,235
Yugoslavia	4,933
Argentina	4,862
Romania	4,588
Colombia	4,464
South Africa	4,084
Australia	4,956
Ethiopia	3,920
China, Taiwan	3,500
Netherlands	3,461
Burma	3,425
Czechoslovakia	3,149
Morocco	2,972
Venezuela	2,912
Saudi Arabia	2,867
North Korea	2,734
Zaire	2,643
Peru	2,580
Sri Lanka	2,527
Algeria	2,450
Greece	2,237
Hungary	2,186
Malaysia	2,139
Chile	2,133
Belgium	2,071
Portugal	2,053

Source: U.S. Bureau of the Census, Kevin Kinsella, Center for International Research, International Data Base

Figure 3

    B. Internationally speaking

        1. In Japan, the life expectancy is greater than 76 years for males and 82 years for females.

        2. A recent international study showed older Americans reported being 'very satisfied' with life, twice as often as the elderly in Japan, and 50% more often than the elderly in Western Germany. -This reported satisfaction is due to the fact that many continue to live in their own homes, rather than with children.

        3. Almost 75% of elderly Americans said they wanted to live in their own homes, even if they were severely disabled.

4. 15% said they would move into an institution, 9% said they would move in with family if necessary.

III. The independent elderly adult

Though we often think of the elderly adult in terms of deterioration, debilitation, and losses, more than 90% of this segment of the population are living independently. They decide when and where to spend their leisure and work times, when to eat, drink, sleep and play. In the last decade there has been an explosion in the field of community organizations and resources for this very active, highly motivated group of individuals. The independent elderly adult tends to have good health, a strong support system, financial security and most importantly, choices.

A. Choosing to retire

1. Considered one of many life transtions, retirement can bring feelings of freedom, independence, or for some financial despair, boredeom and loneliness.

2. Retirement planning often begins very early in one's career, initiating long-term invesments, examining pensions, annuities and setting long-range goals.

3. With sound financial counsel, the retirement years can truly mean a time of rest and relaxation and with good health, it is for many the best years of ones life.

4. For far too many, retirement arrives with the individuals unpreprared for not only the extended years of life, but also realizing that their assets and investments are highly inadequate.

5. For the unprepared, retirement can mean insecurity, dependence on family and frustration with governmental subsidies.

B. Life after retirement

1. As discussed in Chapter 1, retirement may mean an opportunity to start a new career, open a small business, or spend leisurely hours pouring over one's investments.

2. There are a growing number of elderly in the workforce, as mandatory policy regarding retirement disappear. These

individuals want to be productive, appreciated and ease the strain of living on a fixed income.

3. It is predicted that at the turn of the century, the baby boomer generation will be a healthier, better educated population and therefore will delay retirement even longer than today's seniors.

4. McDonald's Corporation has established a program for senior workers over the age of 55, the McMasters program. The effect has been a positive one, stabilizing the work force and increasing productivity.

5. The Regional Coordinating Council for Older Workers is an organization established to assist older adults who wish to remain employed.

6. Senior Corp of Retired Executives (SCORE) has proven to be a powerful organization which utilizes the career experiences of retired adults.

IV. Educational programs for seniors

A. Benefits to seniors

1. Studies confirm that an active mind and an active body lower the risk for mental and physical decline.

2. Universities across the country are seeing an increasing number of senior citizens enrolling in classes, either in pursuit of a degree or for the mere pleasure of advanced learning. For many it is a form of mind-expanding recreation.

3. Professors claim that the older student, those over 65, have insight and experience in the subject matter that is lacking in the younger student. In addition, these seniors are found to be less distractable and more attentive in class.

B. Elderhostel; education and travel

1. Elderhostel, a program which was developed in 1975, provides seniors with a chance to travel, learn and explore the world and meet peers with similar interests and enthusiasm.

- "Elderhostel is for seekers, not for sitters!" explained a manager at one of the many elderhostel campuses.
2. There are elder hostels in all 50 states, 10 Canadian provinces and over 40 countries.
3. The program was designed as a 7-day course within the field of liberal arts, specifically for the senior student.
4. Courses include art, literature, economics and even cross-country skiing.
5. Approximately 200,000 seniors vacation in more than 1200 locations every year.

V. Senior centers

Senior Centers are community gathering places where older persons come together as individuals or groups for services and activities which can enhance their dignity, support their independence and encourage involvement with the neighborhood.

A. Benefits
1. Funded with federal money, these centers provide activities and meals to functional and relatively healthy older adults.
2. Centers offer services for little or no cost, but often take donations to defray operating expenses.
3. Many seniors attend the centers for the hot meals that are provided and the socialization that many crave.
4. Some of the activities include forums on current events, literature review, health promotional topics and assistance with housing and placement decisions.

B. Growth and expansion
1. There are over 10,000 senior centers in the United States which serve approximately one-quarter of the elderly living in the community.
2. Many states mandate senior center development, funding the initiation and expansion of programs.

The Outline Series: Geriatric Nursing -- 43

VI. Transportation services

One of the most difficult decisions an aging individual makes is to relinquish their license to drive. The loss of freedom is usually devastating and is therefore postponed beyong that which is reasonable for physical and cognitive abilities.

A. Losing mobility

1. The effects of aging on vision, perception and judgement are well-documented, yet thousands of accidents occur each year due to an impaired individual behind the wheel.

2. Studies indicate that families are unreliable sources for describing activities of an incompetent driver. To portray the individual as having inadequate judgement and reflexes to operate a vehicle, usually places the burden of transportation on immediate family members, who may be unavailable for such services.

3. For those who have reached the point where driving is no longer feasible, public transportation becomes very vital in keeping close access to the community and its resources.

4. Federal funds have been allocated to provide transportation to those 60 and over through a programn entitled Senior Citizen's Transportation Assistance Program. This service provides a means for seniors who are no longer able to drive or have access to public transportaion the ability to do personal errands, shopping, or attend social engagements.

VII. Adult day care

Adult day care programs were designed to provide respite so that people who would normally qualify for nursing home placement due to a mild impairment to live independently avoid or at least delay being institutionalized. Today, there are millions of older adults living with family who require some form of supervision during the day while the caregiver is either at work, or unavailable to provide 24 hr. care.

A. Supervised care

   1. The first adult day care programs were launched approximately 20 years ago as a service offered by the nursing home industry.

   2. Today there are more than 2500 centers helping over 75,000 impaired elderly persons, responding to the demographic and cultural shift for alternatives to long-term care.

   3. Adult day care centers usually do not accept individuals who are extremely confused or severely handicapped.

   4. Clients need to be able to function somewhat independently, with feeding, toileting, etc., allowing staff to assist minimally in order to preserve independence.

   5. Approximately 40% of the clients have some form of dementia.

B. Services provided within the adult day care setting;

   1. Minimal nursing care

   2. Physical therapy

   3. Dietary therapy

   4. Dispensing of medicine

C. Benefits

   1. Socialization

   2. Recreation and exercise

   3. Meals

   4. Respite for caregivers

   5. The individual who is only mildly cognitively impaired may join discussion groups about current events, literature and other types of educational programs.

   6. The benefits are immeasurable in terms of minimizing decline in physical and interactive skills.

D. Cost of services

   1. The average cost for adult day care may range from $25.00 to $40.00 per day-respite care at home may cost up to $20.00/hr.

   2. Medicaid may pick up the cost for those who are eligible.

   3. Corporations have developed their own programs to assist employees who are struggling with family care issues.

      - Benefits to employers are increased days on the job as well as productivity for workers who have had frequent absences due to the needs of a frail parent.

      - The idea grew out of a survey of employees at IBM corporation after reviewing causes for high absenteeism and distraction among employees.

      - A frequent cause of the problems were related to poor quality or insufficient day care.

   4. The American Business Collaboration for Quality Dependent Care (ABC) exists to improve the infrastructure of child and elder care in local communities.

   5. The movement toward assisting families reflect the widening role of women in the work force.

   6. Statistics show productivity and attendance improve significantly when day care is provided.

E. The daily routine

   A typical day at a center may include breakfast, followed by regularly scheduled health screening, exercise, a brief rest period, a hot lunch, crafts, music, visits from a local Pets for People program and a discussion of current events, movies, or books. The care is individualized, assuring that the clients are given choices, are addressed by the name they wish to be called, and are provided with encouragement and support throughout the day.

46 -- Who are the Elderly

IX. The elderly in the community - volunteer organizations

   A. The typical older volunteer

      1. Older adults who volunteer gain a sense of well-being and improved self-esteem while providing services among the community, utilizing previously gained skills, and maintaining social contacts.

      2. Local organizations in every state are the beneficiary of thousands of hours of labor per year by senior volunteers.

      3. A recent survey found that 9.4 million people over the age of 65 are involved in volunteer work.

   B. Demographics of volunteers

      1. 49% of the population who volunteer are between the ages of 55 and 64

      2. 42% are between the ages of 65 and 74

      3. 27% are over the age of 75

      4. Older volunteers give approximately 5 hrs. per week.

      6. The volunteer hours are spent doing religious work, community service, working with youth and helping with social activities.

      7. One-third of the retired Chief Executive Officers in this country are doing volunteer work in some capacity.

   C. Reasons for doing volunteer work

      1. Desire to do something useful

      2. Enjoyment of the type of work that is done

      3. Hoping to gain some form of new experience or skill

      4. Wanting to benefit a friend or relative

Characteristics of Unpaid Volunteer Workers, by Age Group: May 1989

(numbers of people in thousands)

Characteristic	16+	Age 55-64	65+
Both sexes, total	186,181	21,373	29,153
Unpaid volunteers	38,042	4,455	4,934
As % of total	20.4	20.8	16.9
Men, total	88,656	10,053	12,135
Unpaid volunteers	16,681	1,987	1,917
As % of total	18.8	19.8	15.8
Women, Total	97,525	11,320	17,017
Unpaid volunteers	21,361	2,468	3,016
As % of total	21.9	21.8	17.7
Unpaid volunteers, total	38,042	4,455	4,934
Percent	100.0	100.0	100.0
Type of organization for which work was performed:			
Hospital or other health organization	10.4	12.4	17.8
School or other educational institution	15.1	6.7	4.3
Social or welfare organization	9.9	10.9	14.5
Civic or political organization	13.2	16.1	11.1
Sport or recreation organization	7.8	2.5	1.8
Church or other religious organization	37.4	45.7	43.3
Other organizations	6.3	5.7	7.2
Hours worked per week:			
less than 5 hours	60.0	58.9	53.6
5 to 9 hours	19.9	19.9	23.8
10 to 19 hours	10.8	11.7	11.0
20 to 34 hours	5.8	6.1	7.4
35 hours and over	3.6	3.4	4.2
Median hours worked	4.3	4.4	4.7
Weeks worked per year:			
Less than 5 weeks	20.2	17.5	14.4
5 to 14 weeks	21.2	18.6	16.6
15 to 25 weeks	14.4	12.8	14.8
27 to 49 weeks	15.9	15.9	16.9
50 to 52 weeks	28.3	35.1	37.2
Median weeks worked	25.2	30.5	34.9

SOURCE: U.S. Department of Labor, Bureau of Labor Statistics. "Thirty-Eight Million Persons Do Volunteer Work." Press Release USOL 90-154 (March 29, 1990). Data are from May 1989 Current Population Survey.
NOTE: Data exclude people in institutions.

Figure 4

48 -- Who are the Elderly

Diagram 5. Percent of Adult Population Doing Volunteer Work: 1991
[Covers persons 18 years and over. Volunteers are persons who worked in some way to help others for no monetary pay during the previous year.

AGE, SEX, RACE AND ETHNIC ORIGIN	Percent of population volunteering	Average hours volunteered per week	EDUCATIONAL ATTAINMENT AND HOUSEHOLD INCOME	Percent of population volunteering	Average hours volunteered per week	TYPE OF ACTIVITY	Percent of volunteers involved in activity
Total	51.1	4.2	Elementary school	25.0	(NA)	Arts, culture, humanities	6.2
			Some high school	22.1	5.1	Education	15.4
18-24 years old	48.3	3.2	High school graduate	44.7	4.1	Environment Health	8.6 12.9
25-34 years old	52.9	4.2	Technical, trade, or business school	51.5	3.9	Human services	12.1

The Outline Series: Geriatric Nursing -- 49

AGE, SEX, RACE AND ETHNIC ORIGIN	Percent of population volunteering	Average hours volunteered per week	EDUCATIONAL ATTAINMENT AND HOUSEHOLD INCOME	Percent of population volunteering	Average hours volunteered per week	TYPE OF ACTIVITY	Percent of volunteers involved in activity
45-54 years old	55.9	4.0	Some college	66.1	3.5		
55-64 years old	49.4	4.5	College graduate	76.6	4.6	Informal	23.4
65-74 years old	42.0	4.3				International, foreign	2.3
75 years old and over	26.6	(NA)	Under $10,000	31.6	4.0	Political organizations	4.7
			$10,000-$19,999	37.9	39.	Private, community foundations	2.3
Male	49.2	3.3	$20,000-$29,999	51.3	4.0		
Female	52.9	5.0	$30,000-39,999	56.4	4.7		

AGE, SEX, RACE AND ETHNIC ORIGIN	Percent of population volunteering	Average hours volunteered per week	EDUCATIONAL ATTAINMENT AND HOUSEHOLD INCOME	Percent of population volunteering	Average hours volunteered per week	TYPE OF ACTIVITY	Percent of volunteers involved in activity
			$40,000-$49,999	67.4	4.2	Public and societal benefit	6.4
White	52.6	4.2	$50,000-$59,999	67.7	3.9	Recreation - adults	6.7
Black	43.3	4.5	$60,000-$74,999	55.0	5.1	Religion	26.8
			$75,000-$99,999	62.8	3.7	Work-related organizations	7.1
Hispanic[1]	37.6	4.5	$100,000 or more	73.7	3.7	Youth development	14.7

NA Not available.
[1] Hispanic persons may be of any race.
Source: Hodgkinson, Virginia, Murray Weitzman, and the Gallup Organization, Inc., *Giving and Volunteering in the United States: 1992 Edition*. (Copyright and published by INDEPENDENT SECTOR, Washington, DC, fall 1992.)

X. Health promotion

There are more Americans today involved in health promotion activities than ever before. The number of elderly involved in some form of routine exercise program or rehabilitative routine is also on the increase. Many seniors attack the matter proactively, before disease or debilitation occurs. Others are initiated to the idea of routine exercise after an acute episode of illness, which often includes weight and blood pressure control, or after a surgical repair or possibly trauma, i.e, hip fracture, knee replacement or coronary bypass grafting (CABG.)

A. Types of exercise
1. Today's seniors are avid walkers, using the local enclosed mall, the high school track or just the neighborhood.
2. The YMCA as well as commercial fitness centers report an increase in elder members who enjoy the pool, the track, the weight-training equipment as well as aerobics.
3. Commercial sales of exercise equipment to older Americans has risen significantly in the last decade.

B. Historically
1. Until recently health promotion for seniors was seldom addressed. There has been a paucity of research describing efforts to prevent functional decline and disease.
2. Diet and exercise habits of the 'old old' are studied by researchers hoping to understand the key to longevity and graceful aging.
3. Those that survive into their sunset years, thrive on the challenges of daily living, negotiating the obstacles of aging as optimal health withers.

C. Baseline health
1. Health promotion may require modifying and re-establishing present methods of self care, for alternative coping strategies.
2. Initial assessment of physical, mental and psychosocial functioning allow the health care professional to determine areas of healthy living as well as dysfunction.

D. Health promotion
   1. Components of an effective health promotion program include:
      - Health monitoring on a regular schedule yearly or semi-annually
      - Nutritional review and counseling
      - Establishment of an exercise program
      - Stress management
      - Support through local resources
      - Open discussion of 'end of life' choices
   2. National health promotion efforts:
      - Education/outreach programs which provide information about current health problems, such as arthritis and heart disease. These are often sponsored by local hospitals in a 'public relations' format to enhance public opinion about the institution.
      - Behavioral change seminars which attempt to educate and modify behavior to promote healthier living, i.e. stop smoking, weight loss clinics, stress management.
      - Wellness programs to integrate healthy practices into an individual's lifestyle such as survival skills for widows and widowers, self-defense and effective grandparenting.
      - Medical care instructions which promote becoming more involved in personal health issues, understanding medication interactions, and better comunication methods to deal with your health care providers.
      - Lifesaver classes provide information about preparing for life-threatening emergencies. The 'Vial of Life' and other types of emergency communication systems are explored.
      - Preretirement planning seminars review estate and financial planning topics, drawing up wills, advance directives and other legal issues for seniors.

XI. The elderly adult in transition

It is no surprise that millions of elderly people must give up their independence every year. Often, it is due to debilitation from consequences of the aging process and/or chronic disease, diminished senses, acute illness and even depletion of personal income and assets. Loss of independence is a primary concern at any age, but especially for the older adult, whose chances of resilience and resurgence are lessened. As the life cycle takes yet another turn, role reversal is imminent, as the adult child begins caring for the parent, slowly assuming responsibility for overall physical, emotional and financial care.

A. Role reversal

1. Gradual or abrupt change in typical roles, as the older adult becomes more dependent on immediate family for assistance.

2. The phrase 'Sandwich Generation' has been coined to describe the pressures on today's families to care not only for their own offspring, but also for aging relatives simultaneously.

3. Unfortunately for many, caregivers within the immediate family are not always available, leaving these individuals alone and isolated in the final phase of life.

B. Challenges of aging

1. As health deteriorates and dependency begins, the call for help is initiated.

2. Communities have responded to the needs with extensive resources for both parties; the caregiver and the recipient.

3. Typically, metropolitan areas have bountiful resources available, compared to those found in rural areas.

   - Resources not often found in rural areas; assisted transportation, senior organizations and adult day care centers.

C. Seeking services

1. In most cases, it is the responsibility of the older person to determine the nature of the services needed; where and when to access services as well as appropriate utilization of them.

2. Frustration with the system of senior services is common, leading to either non-use or inappropriate use of them.

3. Cost savings is usually a priority, maximizing dollars from a fixed income in order to utilize and enjoy a variety of opportunities.

XII. Disability

A. Statistically

1. In 1990, about 80% of older persons living in the community had health related difficulties.

2. More than 7 million elderly individuals lost some degree of independent functioning, as measured by the degree of difficulty with activities of daily living. (ADL's)
   - Difficulties with personal needs such as dressing, eating, toileting and personal hygiene
   - Getting around outside the home
   - Doing light housework
   - Preparing meals
   - Managing bills and financial matters

   (See Unit I, Chapter 1, Diagram 9)

3. The risk of functional disability increases rapidly after age 65.

4. The most common difficulty is with walking; the least common is eating.

B. Dealing with disabilities

Studies show a tremendous increase in the number and nature of the rehabilitative and restorative therapies for older adults.

1. Specialty programs within the fields of physical, occupational, and speech therapy have been developed to address areas of dysfunction aggressively.

2. A two-year study of 4,000 older persons living in the community showed a dramatic 25% increased improvement in functional ability after intensive therapeutic involvement.

3. Morbidity, disability and mortality are the most significant issues in geriatrics currently, and will have the greatest impact on research and project development.

XII. Case management

Optimal care for all ages requires proper assessment of not only the existing condition, but also of normal variations from that individual's baseline. The disease processes that accompany aging are frustrating for the client and the health care professional in that many medications, procedures and other by-products of advanced technology have limited value for the elderly person and often cause increased burden without benefit. The case management approach brings together the client, the family and the health care team, working to provide optimal resources.

A. Social workers, nurses, attorneys, financial consultants, and other dedicated professionals have developed specific services which offer guidance and direction for the individual who faces disability.

- The combined team or multi-disciplinary approach blends together the expertise needed to obtain appropriate services and assistance.

B. Case managers are often referred to as 'gatekeepers' or brokers of health care.

C. Case management begins when the family or individual seeks professional help to explore available services and resources for the impaired elderly individual.

- Components of case management include; assessing, planning, coordinating, evaluating and monitoring provision of services.

XIII. Assisted living

Creativity is apparent in the field of transitional housing alternatives for the elderly.

A. ALF (Assisted Living Facility) is a creative housing option, based on a program for the elderly in Sweden.

1. This system utilizes a single-family dwelling, within a neighborhood where anywhere from 5 to 15 older adults live with trained supervisory assistants.

2. Independent activities of daily living are encouraged based on individual abilities and strengths.

3. All the individuals living in the home contribute to the functioning and maintenance of the dwelling, helping with meal preparation, gardening, laundry and daily chores.

4. Currently, there are over 1.5 million residents nationwide living in ALF's.

5. There is no private or federal reimbursement insurance dollars which cover the costs generated from this type of arrangement.

6. Low income elderly, without these assisted types of options, live in subsidized housing projects, without supervision, daily monitoring and support personnel.

B. Retirement communities

1. Another type of assisted living arrangements for singles or couples.

2. Offer a wide menu of services, including transportation, laundry, meals, and social programs.

3. Are usually associated with a nursing care center, should the individual become ill or lose independent functional ability.

4. Costs may range from $20,000 to $200,000 per year

C. ECHO

1. Elder Housing Cottage Opportunity is an economical housing solution which places a small home on the property of a relative to help provide daily supervision and needed assistance.

2. Pilot programs have been funded federally.

3. Restrictied zoning laws may prevent caregivers from exercising this option.

XIV. Caregivers

A. Spouse as caregiver

1. Older adults often rely on their spouse to provide care at home when health begins to deteriorate.

2. Usually the most cost-effective means of providing in-home care

3. Statistically, the caregiver often becomes ill, neglecting their own health in favor of their disabled spouse.

4. Lack of a respite caregiver, such as another relative or friend is the reason most often given for spousal illness.

B. Respite care

1. Respite care is offered to relieve caregivers of an impaired or disabled older adult by providing assistance in the form of a paid caregiver, volunteer, or a family member.

2. Services can be contracted weekly, monthly, or hourly.

3. The Department of Human Services Statewide Respite Program provides up to $2500.00 per year for elder care services.

4. The funds may be used for in-home care, adult day care, or nursing home care.

5. To qualify for the funds, the senior must receive less than $1158.00/mo. and have assets of less than $40,000.

C. Homemakers and home health aides

1. Homemakers and other in-home caregivers are available through private or hospital-based agencies to meet the needs of patients who have been recently discharged from the hospital, or those who consistently are unable to care for themselves.

2. Services include bathing, dressing, light housework, and meal preparation.

3. The fees can range from $10.00 - $20.00 per hour.

58 -- Who are the Elderly

    4. These aides are usually bonded and certified through the Department of Health or accredited by the Commission on Accreditation for Home Care.

    5. Home care aides are frequently trained as a Certified Nurse Aides to provide personal care and other duties as deemed necessary by the specific job description.

XV. Long Term Care

Nursing homes have been by far, the most commonly used facilities for long term care. Currently there are approximately 25,000 nursing homes in this country housing over 1.6 million residents.

  A. The typical nursing home resident:

    1. Female - approximately 75%

    2. Dependent on others for 4 to 5 ADL's

    3. Mostly incontinent - more than 50%

    4. Often mentally impaired - 65%

    5. Often diagnosed with dementia - 43%

    6. Often over the age or 85 - 45%

    7. Receiving rehabilitative services - 50%

    8. Often discharged back to home within a year- 75%

    9. Protected by OBRA regulations since 1987

    10. Provided with the Resident Bill of Rights. (See"Resident's Rights on following pages.)

  B. Wellness/Illness -- The dichotomy

    1. Nursing homes historically have been 'resting grounds' for those with irreversible terminal conditions.

    2. There were relatively few discharges to home after nursing home placement.

    3. One of the primary functions of today's nursing home is to promote wellness, in terms of optimal functioning and quality of life.

Resident's Rights

As a resident you have a right to:

1. **Be fully informed and have free choice.**

   A. To receive a copy of all rules and regulations regarding your rights and responsibilities.

   B. To have a written list of services available and the cost of those services not covered in the facility's rate.

   C. To choose your own doctor, providing the doctor is willing and able to comply with state, federal and facility rules and regulations concerning physician services. This includes regular visits and written notes, orders and exams.

   D. To have your doctor explain your health and medical condition to you unless it is written in your medical record that it is believed not to be in your best interests.

   E. To participate in planning your care and to be fully informed in advance regarding your care and treatment. If you refuse any treatment, you and your responsible party will be told what could happen if you continue to refuse, and this will be written in your medical record. Decisions about the above should be discussed with the patient's doctor so that wishes can be appropriately carried out. In any case, the patient's dignity and comfort will be maintained.

2. **Remain in the facility and have reasonable needs met.**

   A. To be discharged only for medical reasons, non-payment, or for your safety, health and welfare, or that of others, or the facility closes.

   B. To receive services with reasonable allowance for individual needs or preferences beyond what is needed to maintain a safe and orderly facility, i.e. regular meal times, smoking policies, etc.

   C. To be told in advance that your room or roommate is going to be changed and to be involved in a room placement decision as applicable.

Resident's Rights cont.

3. **Voice grievances and exercise rights.**

    A. To express yourself and suggest changes regarding care and treatment or the behavior of other residents, without fear or discrimination, either to facility staff or to outside representatives.

    B. To have concerns and suggestions answered and/or resolved by the facility.

    C. To vote in local, state or federal elections.

    D. You and your family may organize and meet in the facility as a group.

4. **Be free from abuse and restraints.**

    A. To not be given medicine or be restrained without an order from your doctor. If you live in a residential care facility and you are physically restrained any time for any reason, your level of care must be re-evaluated immediately.

    B. To not be physically, mentally, emotionally or sexually injured or harmed.

    C. To not be punished or kept away from others.

    D. To tell anyone from a state or federal agency if you feel you have been abused or neglected. This includes the State Long-Term Care Ombudsman, the Division of Aging, or the Division of Family Services. For information, call 1-800-392-0210.

5. **Confidentiality.**

    A. To not have any information about your medical, personal, social or financial situation shared with any resident or anyone not involved in your care. This information will not be released without your written permission.

6. **Privacy and Respect.**

    A. To be treated with consideration, respect and dignity, including privacy, during treatment and care of your personal needs. (This does not mean you will have a private room.)

    B. To do things for yourself or others, with your doctor's permission, as long as you are able and are not being forced to perform work.

Resident's Rights cont.

7. **Manage your own money.**

   A. To decide who will help manage your personal funds. You may have our facility help you or a family member, friend, responsible party or legal guardian (power of attorney), conservator, etc.

   B. Village North Inc. facilities will hold resident cash funds not to exceed $50.00 for facility residents, You or a guardian/representative will need to sign a permission slip and deposit and/or withdrawal slip at the time of each transaction. A quarterly statement of the balance in your cash fund will be provided.

   If resident cash funds or possessions are not claimed within one year of the resident's departure, this facility will notify the Missouri Department of Social Services for transfer of such funds and possessions to the State Collector of Revenue to escheat to the state of Missouri.

8. **Communicate freely.**

   A. To meet in private with anyone you want, as long as it does not infringe on the rights of another resident.

   B. To make or receive personal calls, with as much privacy as possible.

9. **Participate in activities.**

   A. To attend and participate in social, religious and community activities of your choice, unless your doctor states that it would be harmful or it would infringe on the rights of another resident.

10. **Keep your possessions.**

    A. To keep your clothes or other personal things as space allows.

    B. To have the facility keep a record of all your personal things and have them returned when you leave for any reason.

11. **Marital Privileges.**

    A. To visit with your husband or wife in private.

Resident Rights cont.

  B. To share a room with your husband or wife, if you are both residents, unless one or both of you have a medical condition that makes this impossible, or if one of you does not want to share a room.

12. **Purchase of goods or services.**

  A. To buy or rent anything not included in your daily or monthly charge.

  B. To buy or rent another brand of an item provided in your daily or monthly charge. This includes pharmacy services, but it will be your responsibility to see to it that the medicines needed arrive in a way that meets state, federal and facility rules and regulations regarding pharmacy services.

13. **Examine survey results.**

  A. To see any Medicare or Medicaid survey that lists problems found.

  B. To see the facility's plan to correct these problems. These results are posted on a bulletin board at the nurses station.

14. **Plan of care.**

  A. Since the care of residents is the primary concern of Village North Inc., key professionals and other staff members meet regularly to discuss the individual "Plan of Care" for residents, including treatments, results and goals. Active participation by you and your family members in your "Plan of Care" is encouraged since this cooperation is essential to achieve the best possible results. You will be informed in advance as to the date and time of when your "Plan of Care" is to be discussed.

15. **Patient Bill of Rights and Grievances.**

  A. In providing healthcare services, Village North Inc. assumes the responsibility to place the resident first in all matters relating to the delivery of care. This facility recognizes its obligation to provide the proper care for each resident, as specifically prescribed by the resident's own physician, and to respect the dignity of the resident as a human being. Every resident should expect the highest

Resident Rights cont.

quality of personal and professional treatment and the right to present grievances if the resident feels he/she is not receiving it.

B. If at any time the resident feels he/she has a problem or complaint, procedures for grievances are available. Residents are encouraged to discuss problems with the department supervisor. If resident is not satisfied with the response, he/she should notify the Social Service designee and/or the administrator and request that the problem be investigated and that they assist the resident in a resolution.

C. Even if the resident is not physically or otherwise competent to accept or act upon these rights, they are still the rights of the resident and may be exercised by a guardian or representative on behalf of the resident. Village North Inc. recognizes and fully accepts its professional responsibility to guarantee these rights.

D. No person shall, on the basis of age, sex, race, color, national origin, religion or handicap be denied participation in the services of this facility.

    4. Support systems necessary for rehabilitation and optimal wellness are an integral part of the long term care picture i.e, Physical therapy, Occupational Therapy, etc.

C. Criteria for placement

1. Individuals who have acute or chronic physical or mental impairment which prohibits them from either living independently or is too great a burden to be managed in the home environment.

2. Short term rehabilitative potential which is maximally achieved through the long term care environment and its support services.

3. Hospice patients who choose to have 24 hr. nursing care in a licensed facility rather than at home or in the acute care hospital.

4. Temporary lodging for an impaired individual whose caregiver may need temporary relief from responsibilities.

XVI. Losses

Autonomy is valued by all individuals but especially by those whose independence is imminently diminishing. Once optimal health has disappeared, dependence becomes inevitable. It is important to consider the losses experienced by an older person, who must relinquish independence.

A. The home environment

1. Inability to function as 'head of household'

2. Liquidating assets, including ones lifetime home and furnishings to move into a supervised or assisted environment.

3. Giving up chores to paid service employees i.e. grass cutting, laundry, once physical strength and abilities are diminished.

B. Physical/cognitive abilities

1. Daily activities such as grooming, home and yard work, eating.

2. Impaired cognition limits activities which require accurate memory and thinking, such as bill-paying, grocery shopping, making and keeping appointments and other social activities.

3. Loss of judgement and perception prohibits activities which put lives in danger such as driving a car, operating a lawn mower, using a gas stove or grill, lighting candles or the fireplace.

C. Loss of a spouse

1. Personal losses are immeasurable as one ages.

2. Loss of the spouse immediately requires the remaining individual to assume both roles, in whatever way they have been defined in the marriage.

3. The grief that one endures during the first several years alone often disables the living spouse to the degree that he too becomes dependent.

4. Widowhood may bring about changes in living arrangements, financial status, interactions with social groups as well as isolation.

D. Loss of independence

1. Occurs when one's living arrangements and self-sufficiency are altered either voluntarily or due to the erosion of one's support systems.

2. This may be the watershed event for placement in supervisory care.

3. Activities such as eating, bathing, toileting etc. are at the convenience of the care provider.

4. The impaired individual may experience confusion, combativeness, and noncompliance when placed in unfamiliar surroundings and strange routines.

5. The alert individual who is removed from the home environment and placed in a supervised housing environment, may become depressed, demanding, and agitated as a result of loss of control over body, surroundings, and routine. The reality of these life changes alone can bring about stress, dynsfunctional behavior, and loss of purpose. The goals of health promotion programs for the elderly can't always address the core issues, but rather emphasize stress management and coping mechanisms which may be appropriate for the ongoing transitions.

References

Vierck, Elizabeth. *Fact Book on Aging*, 1990

"Life Here Pretty Good". Philadelphia Inquirer, 9/30/92

Ebersole and Hess. *Toward Healthy Aging*, 1994

U.S. Census Bureau. "Rank of States with 65+ Population"

U.S. Census Bureau. (Countries with more than 2 million elderly in 1991"

U.S. Census Bureau "Counties with more than 2 million elderly in 2020"

U.S. Department of Labor Statistics "Characteristics of Unpaid Volunteers"

Hodgkison, Virginia. Volunteer Work 1991, Independent Sector, "Giving and Volunteering in the U.S."

U.S. Census Bureau "Need for Personal Assistance with Everyday Activities"

Unit 1 - Chapter 3

The Healthy Older American: Assessment of the Geriatric Client

"Health is a state of complete physical, mental and social well-being and not merely the absence of disease or infirmity."

— World Health Organization

The above quote from the World Health Association sets the stage for assessment of the geriatric client. By the age of sixty-five, eighty per cent of older people have at least one chronic disease. But the majority of these seniors live active, healthy lives outside of institutions. While aging frequently does not mean freedom from disease, it does not exclude well-being. Appropriate health care for the aging individual should promote physical, mental and social well-being despite the many changes that are taking place.

Aging alters the older adult's response to disease. Generally, the problems that affect older adults are expressions and combinations of physical, social and psychological problems which can combine to have an unhealthy effect on the individual and his family. As a result, the need for comprehensive assessment of physical, psychological, social and functional capabilities and disabilities is critical in order to plan interventions that will be individualized and effective. The ultimate goal is to encourage active and productive aging which will promote optimal quality of life.

Many nurses will function as part of an interdisciplinary team whose goals are to assess and manage the geriatric client. While nurses may not always perform all components of the geriatric assessment, it is important to understand each of the pieces and their implications;

This chapter will outline six parts of the geriatric assessment:

    I.   History

    II.   Functional assessment

    III. Psychosocial assessment

    IV. Cognitive assessment

    V.   Physical Examination

    VI. Laboratory tests

Components of the Complete Geriatric Assessment

Components of the Assessment Key Areas for Assessment
Health History Medical History

Medications, Allergies

Health Habits

Health Maintenance

Review of Systems--Functional Assessment Activities of Daily Living

Bathing, Dressing, Eating, Mobility

Transfers, Continence

Instrumental Activities of Daily Living

Shopping, Housekeeping, Cooking

Finances, Transportation, Medications,

Telephone--Psychosocial Assessment Meaningful Activity

Relationships

Mental Health

Financial/Planning Issues--Mental Status Assessment History of Changes

Mental Status Testing--Physical Examination Complete Physical Examination

Identification of Normal Aging Changes   vs. Abnormal Findings

Laboratory Studies

FIGURE 1

Key issues for assessing the older adult will be discussed, sample forms and standardized assessment tools presented.

I. **Underlying principles used when assessing the older client:**

   A. Misunderstanding of normal aging

   1. Patients and health professionals may have little knowledge about normal aging.

   2. Historically this has resulted in under-reporting of symptoms which are thought to be normal with age.

   - For example, older women often think that incontinence is the result of aging and may fail to report it to their doctor. In fact, a number of treatment options exist and 70% of incontinence problems can be improved if not cured.

   B. Multiple chronic diseases

   1. The presence of more than one condition can confuse the assessment, as symptoms can often be caused by more than one disease.

   2. It can take some detective work to sort out the cause and effect of current problems.

   C. Multiple Medications

   1. Most adults take multiple prescription medications.

   2. The potential for side effects, interactions and toxicity can relate to the client's symptoms or problems and should be explored thoroughly.

   D. Altered presentation of illness

   1. The elderly client may have different signs and symptoms of disease than the younger client.

   2. They are likely to present with functional symptoms of illness such as confusion, falls or fatigue. Classic symptoms such as chest pain in the event of a heart attack or fever in an infection may be muted in the elderly client making it easy to miss a diagnosis.

HISTORY

II. Overview

The purpose of the history is to identify current lifestyle and health problems, significant past medical illnesses which may impact current health and symptomatology which may indicate disease. The older adult has a long history and it is important to focus on the relevant points during the interview. It is essential to conserve time and energy to avoid fatigue and frustration in the elderly client.

A. Develop a history from which notes past illnesses, surgeries and a symptom checklist to help frame the interview (See sample - the client can fill this out prior to the interview).

- Avoid general questions which may elicit non-specific symptoms such as "hurting all over", weakness, etc. Vague symptoms such as fatigue are common. Ask specific questions about when the symptoms occur, severity, frequency and any precipitating factors such as activity and time of day.

B. Interview a collateral source, i.e. a spouse, adult child, or a close friend privately to confirm and gather additional information when possible. This is especially important if you suspect a memory problem.

C. Assessment of medications should include the use of prescription medications, all PRN and over-the-counter drugs, as well as vitamins and supplements. Ask the patient to bring all of their medications in for the assessment if possible. Check for compliance by counting the number of pills and comparing with the date and number dispensed by the pharmacy (written on prescription).

D. Deficits in vision and hearing are common. The environment should be free of background noise and have adequate lighting.

E. The client may tire easily, so be concise and take a break midway through the interview if necessary.

F. Maintain the client's dignity and address them by their last name. Let them know what will be happening as you proceed. (Note: a client with advanced memory loss may not recognize their own last name, in which case the first name would be more familiar.)

III. Key areas for assessment:

A. Medical history:

1. What is the reason for seeking care?

2. Describe past illnesses?

3. Were there any hospitalizations (if applicable)? Where?

4. Explain any surgeries?

B. Medications:

1. What medications does the individual take? (Include such things as vitamins, aspirin, laxatives, lotions and creams, eye drops, and any over-the-counter medications).

2. Why is each medication taken?

3. When is the medication taken? What happens if a dose is missed?

C. Allergies:

1. Have there been any allergic reactions to medicine?

    - What was the medication and what type of reaction?

    - Are there any other allergies?

D. Smoking

1. Does the client currently smoke cigarettes, cigars, a pipe?

2. How many years have they smoked?

3. How many packs were smoked per day?

4. When did they last smoke?

5. Have there been any health problems because of smoking?

E. Immunizations:

Have they had the following immunizations:

1. Pneumonia vaccine (one time after age 65)?

2. Flu shot (yearly)?

3. Tetanus shot (every 10 years)?

4. Were there any adverse reactions to immunizations?

F. General Health Indicators:

1. How would they rate their present health: excellent, good, fair or poor?

2. Has the individual gained or lost weight in the past year? How much?

3. Does the client have any trouble sleeping? Waking up or getting to sleep?

G. Review of Systems:

1. Overview of symptoms related to the various systems (see sample form)

2. Gastrointestinal

3. Genitourinary

4. Skin

5. Sensory

6. Pulmonary

7. Cardiovascular

8. Endocrine

9. Nervous

10. Musculoskeletal

Washington University Division of Geriatrics

PRELIMINARY HEALTH HISTORY FORM

(Sample Form ...This can be sent to the client prior to the office visit to save time.)

These questions are an important part of your health history. Please fill this out and bring it with you to the doctor. If someone else is filling out the form, please answer for the patient to the best of your ability.

Patient Name _____ Date _____

Date of Birth _____ Age _____

Marital Status:

   Single ___ Married ___ Separated ___ Divorced ___ Widowed ___

Insurance:

   Medicare ___ Medicaid ___ Other: _____

Highest Grade Completed in School: _____

Type of Residence:

   House ___ Apartment ___ Nursing Home ___ Other _____

Person Completing Form _____

Relationship to Patient _____

Phone _____

Reason for Appointment _____

_____

Who are your doctors? (List primary care doctor first)

_____

_____

Have you had any illnesses or hospitalizations? Please list.

_____

_____

_____

Have you had any operations? List the date and type of surgery.

_____

_____

_____

_____

What medications do you take? (Include such things as vitamins, aspirin, laxatives) *PLEASE BRING ALL YOUR MEDICINES WITH YOU*

NAME	FREQUENCY	DOSE

Have you ever had an allergic reaction to a medicine?

Yes _____ No _____

If yes, what kind? _____

Do you have any other allergies? _____

_____

Do you currently smoke cigarettes?

Yes _____ No _____ Packs/day _____

Have you ever smoked cigarettes on a daily basis?

Yes _____ No _____ Packs/day _____

Total number of years smoked _____

Date of last use _____

Other tobacco use: Yes _____ No _____

Immunizations: (Fill in date last received)

    Flu shot _____ Tetanus shot _____

    Pneumonia shot _____ Tuberculosis test _____

How would you rate your present physical health?

    Excellent ____ Good ____ Fair ____ Poor ____

Do you have trouble falling asleep or waking up at night?

    Yes ____ No ____

Have you lost or gained weight in the past year?

    Yes ____ No ____

How many days a week do you exercise? _____

What type? _____

SYMPTOM REVIEW

	YES	NO
Have you had a change in your appetite?	___	___
Have you had any change in your bowel movements in the past year?	___	___
Have you ever had blood in your stool or tarry looking stools?	___	___
Have you ever had yellow jaundice or hepatitis?	___	___
Do you ever have heartburn or indigestion?	___	___
Do you ever have pain in your stomach or abdomen?	___	___
Have you ever had an ulcer?	___	___
Have you ever had gallbladder problems?	___	___
Have you ever had polyps in your colon or colon cancer?	___	___
Have you ever had a colonoscopy or sigmoidoscopy?	___	___
Is constipation a problem for you?	___	___
Do you ever lose control of your bowels?	___	___

	Yes	No
Do you get up more than twice at night to urinate?	___	___
Do you have to urinate frequently during the day?	___	___
Does your urine burn or hurt when you urinate?	___	___
Do you ever lose control of your bladder or leak urine?	___	___
Have you ever had a kidney stone?	___	___
Have you had a kidney or bladder infection in the past year?	___	___
Do you have any problems with sexual relations?	___	___
Have you ever had syphilis or "bad blood?"	___	___
(For men..)Have you had problems with your prostate?	___	___
Do you have any skin sores that have not healed?	___	___
Have you found any large glands or lumps on your body?	___	___
Are you troubled by a skin rash or itching?	___	___
Do you have trouble hearing people speak to you?	___	___
Have you had a recent change with your vision?	___	___
Has your voice changed or become hoarse?	___	___
Do you get short of breath easily?	___	___
Do you have a cough when you don't have a cold?	___	___
Have you ever had asthma?	___	___
Have you ever had an abnormal chest x-ray?	___	___
Have you ever been told you have a heart murmur?	___	___
Do you sleep propped up or wake up short of breath?	___	___
Do you ever have pain or discomfort in your chest, neck or arms?	___	___
Do you have swelling of the ankles?	___	___

	Yes	No
Do you have fevers or night sweats?	——	——
Have you ever taken medicine for a thyroid problem?	——	——
Have you ever had trouble with your blood?	——	——
Do you bleed or bruise easily?	——	——
Have you had any slurring of your speech?	——	——
Do you have frequent or severe headaches?	——	——
Do you ever get dizzy or lightheaded?	——	——
Have you ever passed out or lost consciousness?	——	——
Do you have problems or changes in your memory?	——	——
Do you often feel unhappy or depressed?	——	——
Have you ever been treated for psychiatric or nervous condition?	——	——
Do you have any joint pains or arthritis?	——	——
Do you have night cramps?	——	——
Do you have cramps in your legs when you walk?	——	——
Have you ever had a back injury?	——	——
Do you have back pain regularly?	——	——
Have you fallen during the last 12 months?	——	——
Have you hurt yourself in a fall?	——	——
Have you ever had a hip fracture?	——	——
Do you have any difficulty walking or with your balance?	——	——
Are you fearful of falling?	——	——

For women:

Have you had change of life (menopause)? If yes, at what age? _____	——	——
Have you had a hysterectomy?	——	——

Have you ever had breast cancer? ___ ___

Have you ever taken female hormones (estrogen)? ___ ___

When was your last pelvic exam and Pap test? _____

Do you have a discharge from your vagina? ___ ___

When was your last breast X-ray (mammogram)? _____

Do you have any lumps or discharge from your breasts? ___ ___

Interpretation:

Any positive responses on the Preliminary Health History should be explored with the client as to duration and frequency of symptoms, treatments that may or may not work, prior evaluation or treatment.

IV. Nursing implications:

A. The health history

1. Identify positive or negative health habits such as exercise, smoking, etc. Use the information to plan education or interventions to promote a healthier lifestyle for the individual.

2. Identify health maintenance problems.

3. Does the individual have a primary care practitioner?

4. Do they understand any health problems or medications?

5. Have the appropriate screening tests been performed such as cancer screening (mammogram and PAP test for women or prostate testing and examination for men)?

   - Education regarding screening tests or health management can help the client take charge of their health.

6. Identify current or past symptoms or illnesses for follow up and further evaluation and exploration on the physical examination.

B. Functional Assessment

The purpose of the functional assessment is to evaluate independence in daily activities and management of the home environment. Independent functioning is one of the main concerns of older adults in managing their health and one of the most important issues in planning nursing care.

1. Chronic medical problems result in reduction of functional ability and the opposite can also be true; functional problems can interfere with the management of disease. As a result, evaluation of functional abilities should always be a part of the geriatric assessment.

   - Determine the client's current level of functioning. When there are deficits, identify when and why changes have occurred.
   - Determine if the changes are related to physical problems or difficulty with memory or thinking. (Confirm findings with collateral source.)
   - When deficits are present, determine whether compensatory mechanisms are in place, the use of supportive services, etc.
   - Functional assessment can be attained through questioning or observation of performance measures. Some of these measures can be incorporated into the assessment:

   a. The patient's ability to undress and dress for the examination

   b. Observation of walking

   c. Ability to follow instructions
      - Use a collateral source to provide input and confirm findings.
      - Consider male and female roles for this generation when assessing functional abilities such as household chores. For example, men may have never been responsible for cooking or house work; women may not have handled finances.

Instruments

The OARS (Older American Resource and Services Center Instrument, 1974) is one example of a standardized measurement of basic and instrumental activities of daily living. Standardized, scored instruments are useful in tracking changes and improvements and in evaluating the outcomes of treatment such as surgery, therapy or medications. The OARS provides clinical information for assessing needs and planning interventions.

Other instruments that are commonly used include the Katz Index of Activities of Daily Living (1963), the dBarthel Index (1979) and the Lawton Scale for Instrumental Activities of Daily Living (1969).

Key Areas for Assessment:

A. Basic Activities of Daily Living (BADLs)

Activities of Daily Living refer to personal care issues, and have been called "those things Mother used to do for you." They require the most intensive help when deficits are present. The following are questions to ask when assessing the following areas:

Eating:
- Can the individual eat independently?
- Are they able to use all utensils?
- Do they need assistance with special preparations, serving or cutting?
- Do they need adaptive equipment?
- Is there difficulty with chewing, swallowing or dentures?
- Can they care for dentures or equipment without help?
- If help is needed, who provides it?

Mobility:
- Does the individual have difficulty with walking and balance?
- Are they able to ambulate independently?
- Is there a walking aid and is it used properly?
- Have they fallen or is there fear of falling such that it interferes with daily activities?

Transfers:
- Is the individual able to get in and out of bed without assistance?
- Is there adaptive equipment needed?
- Can they transfer from chair or toilet?

Continence:
- Does the individual have difficulty with leaking or losing control of bladder or bowels?
- What is the history of symptoms, frequency and amount?
- How is it handled?
- Do they use incontinence products?
- Is a colostomy or urostomy present?

Bathing:
- Does the individual need assistance with bathing or reminders to bathe?
- What kind of bath does the person take? (If the individual is taking only sponge baths, is it because of functional difficulty getting in and out of the bathtub? Is there a shower available?)
- Are there safety issues such as no-slip mats or grab rails for getting in and out of the tub?

Dressing:
- Is the individual physically able to get dressed?
- Can they reach socks and shoes, handle buttons, zippers, snaps?
- Are they able to pick out appropriate clothes?
- Are clothes put on correctly?
- Are reminders needed that clothes are soiled?

B. **Instrumental Activities of Daily Living (IADLs)**

Instrumental Activities of Daily Living are more complex tasks than the BADLS. These have been referred to as "Those things you need to be able to do to move out on your own," or to maintain independent living.

Housekeeping and Laundry:
- Is the individual able to keep their home clean?
- Can they handle laundry and yard work without help?
- If not the primary housekeeper, does the individual participate at all in cleaning or housework or yard work? What are the problems?
- If help is required, how is it provided?

Cooking:
- Is the individual able to cook?
- If not the primary cook, can a light meal be prepared?
- What are the problems with cooking?
- Are there dietary restrictions? How is this observed?

Groceries and shopping:
- Does the individual shop for groceries or other essential items?
- If not the primary shopper, is the individual able to do any shopping or pick up items independently?
- Are they able to get other shopping needs met such as medications, clothes, etc.?

Finances:
- Can the individual handle money, pay bills, write checks or balance the checkbook? - Does anyone oversee their finances or checkbook?
- What are the problems?

Transportation:
- Is the individual able to get places independently?
- Are they able to drive or use other kinds of transportation?
- Have there been any safety problems or accidents, such as getting lost?
- What kind of assistance is needed?

Medication:
- Is the individual able to take medications independently?
- Is there any system for remembering to take medications?
- Are reminders necessary?
- Have their been problems taking medications?
- What are the problems?

Telephone:
- Is the individual able to use the phone without help?
- Are there related hearing or visual deficits?
- Able to look up or remember numbers?
- Explain how to access emergency help?

OARS Activities of Daily Living and Instrumental Activities of Daily Living

A. Activities of Daily Living

Score   Description

1. Can you eat . . .
   - 2   Without help (able to feed yourself completely,
   - 1   With some help (need help with cutting, etc.),
   - 0   Or, are you completely unable to feed yourself?

_____ Score

2. Can you walk . . .
   - 2   Without help (except from a cane),
   - 1   With some help (from a person, use of a walker, crutches, etc.),
   - 0   Or are you completely unable to walk?

_____ Score

3. Can you get in and out of bed . . .

   2   Without any help or aids,

   1   With some help (either from a person or with the aid of some device),

   0   Or are you totally dependent on someone else to lift you?

_____ Score

4. Do you ever have trouble getting to the bathroom on time?

   2   No

   1   Have catheter or colostomy

   0   Yes - have incontinence

_____ Score

5. Can you take a bath or shower . . .

   2   Without help,

   1   With some help (need help getting in and out of the tub, or need special attachments on the tub),

   0   Or are you completely unable to bathe yourself?

_____ Score

6. Can you dress and undress yourself . . .

   2   Without help (able to pick out clothes, dress and undress yourself),

   1   With some help,

   0   Or are you completely unable to maintain your appearance yourself?

_____ Score

_____ **Total ADL Score**

B. **Instrumental Activities of Daily Living**
   1. Can you do your housework . . .
      - 2 Without help (can scrub floors, etc.),
      - 1 With some help (can do light housework, but need help with heavy work),
      - 0 Or are you completely unable to do any housework?

   _____ Score

   2. Can you prepare your own meals . . .
      - 2 Without help (plan and cook full meals yourself,
      - 1 With some help (can fix simple meals or heat up food, but unable to cook all meals),
      - 0 Or are you completely unable to do any cooking?

   _____ Score

   3. Can you go shopping for groceries . . .(Assuming you have transportation)
      - 2 Without help (take care of all shopping needs yourself, assuming you had transportation),
      - 1 With some help (need someone to go with you on all shopping trips),
      - 0 Or are you completely unable to do any shopping?

   _____ Score

   4. Can you handle your own money . . .
      - 2 Without help (write checks, pay bills, etc.),
      - 1 With some help (manage day to day but need help with managing your checkbook and paying your bills),
      - 0 Or are you completely unable to handle money?

   _____ Score

5. Can you get to places out of walking distance . . .
   - 2 Without help (can travel alone on buses, taxis, or drive yourself),
   - 1 With some help (need someone to help you or go with you when traveling),
   - 0 Or are you unable to travel unless special arrangements are made for a specialized vehicle such as an ambulance?

_____ Score

6. Can you take your medications . . .
   - 2 Without help (in the right doses at the right time),
   - 1 With some help (able to take medicine if someone prepares it for you and/or reminds you to take it),
   - 0 Or are you completely unable to take your medications?

_____ Score

7. Can you use the telephone . . .
   - 2 Without help (including looking up numbers and dialing),
   - 1 With some help (can answer the phone or dial the operator in an emergency, but need special phone or help in getting the number or dialing),
   - 0 Or are you completely unable to use the telephone?

_____ Score

_____ Total IADL Score

_____ Total ADL Score

_____ Overall Score

Interpretation:

Scoring allows the health care professional to evaluate abilities and problems with function in each area. It is also important to identify what support systems the client has for meeting these daily needs. The higher the score, the more independent the client is in daily activities, with a maximum score of 26. A lower score indicates the need for more assistance with daily activities, a score of O indicates total dependence. Lower scores are associated with the need for nursing home placement, and more dependence in the basic activities of daily living often results in a move to a more supportive environment.

Nursing Implications:

Results of the functional assessment can assist the nurse in the following ways:

1. To plan interventions specific to each patient's abilities and promote rehabilitation for abilities that have changed:
   - Monitor changes or improvement in abilities with treatment or interventions or to prior functional status,
   - Direct referrals for rehabilitation: physical therapy (muscle strengthening, assistive devices such as a cane or walker), occupational therapy (adaptive equipment such as for bathing or dressing), speech therapy (swallowing or communication improvement) or patient education (medication management, foot care),
   - Identify what abilities are needed for the client to return home or to prior environment,
2. To identify the level of care needed at time of discharge (from hospital, rehabilitation or home care). When deficits exist, the potential for moving to a more supportive environment is based on the ability of the family/community to provide the services needed to make up for client deficits. Arrangements for care can include:
   - Continue current situation (either independently or with current assistance)
   - Continue current situation with additional family/community support services
   - Assisted living (usually provide supportive services during the day only)
   - 24 hour care such as a nursing home

and presence of mental health problems. A few of the basic tenets to keep in mind:

- The changes and losses common in later life increase the older adult's risk for loneliness, isolation and depression. Adjustment is required for the many changes which can occur: retirement, widowhood, moving, loss of friends, decreased income, declining health.

- Basic personality characteristics tend to be stable throughout adult life, including the later years. The ability to adapt and change remain, although the support systems to help the individual through these changes may be diminished.

- The ethnic background should serve as a context for the assessment with cultural values and differences taken into account.

- Educational level is usually much lower for the older adult i.e, less than 12 years of formal education.

Instruments

- The OARS (Older American Resource Center Instrument) measure of Social Resources is an example of a standardized measure of social functioning.

- The short form of the Geriatric Depression Scale is a brief screening instrument for depression. Depression is common in older adults, especially in those that are hospitalized and is underdiagnosed. Depression is common in the elderly; elderly men have one of the highest rate of suicide. Other scales commonly used for assessment of depression in the elderly include the Hamilton, or the Beck Depression Scales.(1972)

Key Areas for Assessment

A. Meaningful Activity and Relationships

The following questions provide a significant measure of the client's social network and social support. Review answers with collateral source for collaboration.

Activities and Recreation:

- Does the individual engage in any meaningful activity such as work, volunteering, church or social organizations?

- Are there any hobbies or interests?
- Are there any difficulties with these?

Typical Day:

- Describe a typical day.
- How is it divided in terms of self-care, work (or housework) and leisure?
- Is there opportunity for spending time alone and time with others?

Family/significant others:

- Who are the immediate family members and what is the family history?
- How is the marital relationship?
- Are there social contacts? (may include neighbors, friends, co-workers, etc.)
- Is there a confidante?
- Are there problems with sexuality?
- Is there possible elder abuse?

Living situation:

- Does the individual live alone or with others?
- Is there someone available for assistance?
- Are there financial constraints for outside assistance if needed?
- Are there any difficulties?

Roles and responsibilities:

- What is their current involvement in relationships or activities?
- Are there any changes or problems?
- Have there been recent losses?
- Is there dependence on others for care and assistance?
- Are children or others dependent on them?

B. Mental Health

Explore whether or not the client is experiencing any mental health problems, or has a history which might increase their risk of future mental health problems, such as depression, anxiety, paranoia.

History or current mental health problems:

- Is there any history of psychiatric or mental health problems such as anxiety, depression, problems with nervousness or difficulty sleeping?
- Did the individual ever receive treatment and was it helpful?
- Are there current difficulties?
- What are the symptoms and severity of the problem?
- Are there any suicidal thoughts?

Drug/alcohol abuse:

- Is there a problem with alcohol or drug abuse?
- Is there a problem among family members?

Issues and coping mechanisms:

- Are there many changes or losses?
- How is the individual coping with these?
- Are there any particular stressors which the person or family is dealing with?
- What are their coping mechanisms and resources?
- Are their spiritual supports/issues?

Sleep disorders:

Though sleep patterns for the individual change with age, sleep disorders are not only frustrating, but may lead to decreased functioning due to day-time drowsiness. Included in the normal changes in sleep patterns are:

- 'Lighter', shorter periods of sleep
- Decreased periods of 'deep' sleep
- Frequent nap periods

Questions regarding sleep disorders include:
- Nature, onset, duration of sleep problem
- Snoring, severity, and sleep apnea
- Unusual body movements during sleep
- Daytime drowsiness
- Family history of sleep disorders
- Insomnia
- Waking up early and not being able to return to sleep
- Use of medications
- Psychiatric history

C. **Financial/Planning Issues**:

Determine the clients financial status and planning for future health, financial or retirement changes.

Income:
- What are the sources of income?
- Are there difficulties?
- Will retirement provide for current lifestyle?
- Is lack of income affecting their nutrition or ability to pay for medical care, medications, or creating other health issues?

Health Insurance:
- Does the individual have insurance?
- Is it adequate?
- Is there long term care insurance?

Advance directives:
- Does the individual have written advance directives?
- Are there instructions regarding extent of care the person would want in case of a catastrophic illness?
- Is there an appointed surrogate if unable to speak for themselves?
- Can family or a responsible party access money or information in case the individual is unable to do so?

OARS SOCIAL RESOURCE SCALE

1. Are you:

   ____ Single

   ____ Married

   ____ Widowed

   ____ Divorced

   ____ Separated

2. Who lives with you:

   ____ No one

   ____ Husband or wife

   ____ Children

   ____ Grandchildren

   ____ Parents

   ____ Brothers and sisters

   ____ Other relatives

   ____ Friends

   ____ Non-related paid helper

   ____ Other:_____

3. How many people do you know well enough to visit with in their homes?

   ____ Five or more

   ____ Three to four

   ____ One or two

   ____ None

4. About how many times did you talk to someone -- friends, relatives, or others on the telephone in the past week (either you called them or they called you)?

   ____ Once daily or more

   ____ 2-6 times

   ____ Once

   ____ Not at all

5. How many times during the past week did you spend time with someone who does not live with you (either you went to see them, or they came to see you?)

   ____ Once daily or more

   ____ 2-6 times

   ____ Once

   ____ Not at all

6. Do you have someone you can trust and confide in?

   ____ Yes

   ____ No

7. Do you find yourself feeling lonely?

   ____ Quite often

   ____ Sometimes

   ____ Almost never

8. Do you see your relatives and friends?

   ____ As often as you want to

   ____ You are unhappy about how little you see them

9. Is there someone who would give you help if you were sick or disabled?

   ____ Yes

   ____ No

10. Is there someone who could take care of you:

   ____ As long as needed (indefinitely)

   ____ For a short time (a few weeks to months)

   ____ Now and then (fixing lunch, taking to doctor)

Interpretation:

Scoring: Evaluate answers and select the category below that best describes help available and the quality of the social network, based on the above questions.

____**Excellent social resources**: Social relationships are very satisfying and extensive; at least one person would take care of her (him) indefinitely.

____**Good social resources**: Social relationships are fairly satisfying and adequate and at least one person would take care of her (him) indefinitely (or)

____**Social relationships** are very satisfying and extensive, and only short-term help is available.

____**Mildly socially impaired**: Social relationships are unsatisfactory, of poor quality, few; but at least one person would take care of her(him) indefinitely; (or)

____**Social relationships** are fairly satisfactory and adequate, and only short-term help is available.

____**Moderately socially impaired**: Social relationships are unsatisfactory, of poor quality, few; and only short-term care is available (or)

____ **Social relationships** are at least adequate or satisfactory, but help would only be available now and then.

____**Severely socially impaired**; Social relationships are unsatisfactory, of poor quality, few; and help would be available only now and then.(or)

____**Social relationships** are at least satisfactory or adequate, but help is not available, even now and then.

____**Totally socially impaired**: Social relationships are unsatisfactory, of poor quality; and help is not available, even now and then.

GERIATRIC DEPRESSION SCALE (SHORT FORM)

Answer yes or no to each of the following questions. Choose the answer that best describes the way you have felt over the past week:

		Yes	No
1.	Are you basically satisfied with your life?	___	___
2.	Have you dropped many of your activities and interests?	___	___
3.	Do you feel that your life is empty?	___	___
4.	Do you often get bored?	___	___
5.	Are you in good spirits most of the time?	___	___
6.	Are you afraid that something bad is going to happen to you?	___	___
7.	Do you feel happy most of the time?	___	___
8.	Do you often feel helpless?	___	___
9.	Do you prefer to stay at home, rather than going out and doing new things?	___	___
10.	Do you feel you have more problems with memory than most?	___	___
11.	Do you think it is wonderful to be alive now?	___	___
12.	Do you feel pretty worthless the way you are now?	___	___
13.	Do you feel full of energy?	___	___
14.	Do you feel that your situation is hopeless?	___	___
15.	Do you think that most people are better off than you are?	___	___

Interpretation:

    Score _____

Scoring: Add up all bolded answers. A higher score indicates more depressive symptoms. A score of 5 or greater suggests depression and should be evaluated. Refer the patient to their physician or counselor.

Nursing Implications:

The assessment of the clients psychosocial situation will assist in identifying community resources and interventions:

- Inadequate support systems may be improved by gaining the involvement of family, friends, neighbors, a geriatric case manager or other social service agencies which will coordinate care and provide or obtain assistance as needed. The Division of Aging may be called in for services or situations of elder abuse or neglect, or clients needing guardianship.

- Counseling or mental health services may be indicated for the individual with adjustment problems, depression or other mental illness, drug or alcohol abuse. Support groups for individuals with various illnesses or problems are often available through local churches, hospitals or voluntary organizations. Widow's support groups and support groups for people with pulmonary problems, cancer or arthritis are some examples.

- Referral to services which offer activity and recreation, education and opportunity for socialization. Some examples include senior centers, adult day care programs, AARP (American Association of Retired Persons), OASIS (Older Adult Service and Information System), Elderhostel.

- The client's living situation may be contributing to their isolation or boredom. An environment where people, services and activities are available might improve their quality of life. Congregate living situations often provide these options and can include retirement centers or senior housing.

MENTAL STATUS ASSESSMENT

Overview

The purpose of the mental status testing is to determine possible cognitive loss. Because the incidence of Alzheimer's Disease and memory loss increase with age (over 50% in those over 85), formal evaluation of mental status should be a routine part of every assessment. Memory problems are not readily picked up during the interview when changes are mild. Social skills are often maintained and used to cover memory loss.

- Normal changes in memory with age result in less efficiency in learning new information and the process of recall is slower. These changes require more effort to learn new information but should not effect daily activities.

- Testing of memory can be stressful as those with memory loss may try to cover up for deficits.

- Presenting the testing as a routine part of the assessment will almost always result in acceptance. Introduce the testing as having some easy and hard questions.

Instruments

- The Short Blessed Test of Orientation - Memory -Concentration: (Katzman, 1983) One of the quickest screening tests for identifying cognitive impairment.

- Other commonly used screening tests for memory include the Mini-Mental State Examination (Folstein, Folstein and McHugh, 1975 and the Short Portable Mental Status Questionnaire (Pfeiffer, (1975).

Key Areas for Assessment

General Orientation Questions:

- Is the person oriented to person, place and time?
- Have there been periods of confusion?

Identification of Change in Memory and Thinking:

- Have there been changes in memory over time?
- Does the person have difficulty with daily activities because of problems with memory and thinking?

Short Blessed Test of Orientation-Memory-Concentration

Question	Maximum Errors	Error x Weight = Score
1. What year is it now?	1	____ x 4= ____
2. What month is it now?	1	____ x 3= ____

Repeat this phrase after me and remember it:

John Brown 42 Market Street, Chicago

3. About what time is it? (within 1 hour)	1	____ x 3= ____
4. Count backwards from 20 to 1.	2	____ x 2= ____
5. Say the months of the year in reverse order.	2	____ x 2= ____
6. Repeat the name and address I asked you to remember (circle any correct):		
John Brown, 42 Market Street, Chicago	5	____ x 2= ____

Scoring: A score of 0-7 is within the normal limits of changes in memory with age. A score of 8 or greater suggests cognitive impairment and the maximum score is 24. Those with mild memory loss may still score within the normal range. The test is not diagnostic for the cause of the memory loss and the client should be evaluated further. If memory loss is suspected and collateral informants have noticed a change in memory and thinking, it may still be appropriate to refer the patient for further evaluation, even if they score within the normal range.

Nursing Implications:

Evaluation of cognitive impairment is important as some causes are reversible including medications, nutritional deficiencies, thyroid problems and other medical causes. New research is leading to possible medications to treat Alzheimer's disease so that early identification of problems may hold opportunity for slowing if not arresting or improving the disease. The client may need to be followed over time to evaluate changes in memory or thinking. In addition, services and supports for the memory impaired client can improve their quality of life and prevent complications, even if nothing can be done to treat the disease.

Physical assessment

The purpose of the physical assessment is to determine alterations which could indicate disease. This review will not cover all of the physical examination, but will discuss common findings in the older adult and its relevance. For a complete review of physical examination, see Leukenotte, 1991, Bates, or other comprehensive guide to physical assessment.)

The aging process results in decreased efficiency in functioning for most of the organ systems. However, these changes should not cause disability in the absence of disease. The resulting loss of reserves does make the older adult at risk for more severe reactions to illness, stress and trauma.

- Normal aging changes are those changes which are universal; all people will experience them to some degree if they live long enough. Examples of normal changes are wrinkles and gray hair.

- Normal aging changes may occur at varying rates in individuals, and there can be wide variation from person to person. Some people develop gray hair in their twenties or earlier, others in their fifties. One individual may have gray hair, but few wrinkles in their sixties.

- Genetic and environmental factors, such as exposure to sunlight or deconditioning can combine to effect the rate of aging changes and likelihood of disease.

Key areas for assessment:

Inspection and palpation of the head and neck

Eyes:

- Are the pupils slow or slightly unequal in reacting to light? This can result in the older adult needing more light to see well, difficulty seeing at night and slower adjustment when moving from light to dark rooms.

- Are there difficulties differentiating colors such as blue/green/violet? A yellowing of the lens can lead to changes in color perception.

- Does the external eye show evidence of conjunctivitis, entropion or ectropion; (turning of the eyelids inward or outward) that might interfere with vision?
- Are they able to read newsprint (test vision with and without glasses)? Can they see objects across the room?
- Do they have appropriate glasses? Are there problems with peripheral vision suggesting glaucoma?
- Does the fundoscopic exam show an absence of the red reflex which may suggest cataracts? Is there evidence of papilledema, arterial narrowing, exudates or increased vascularization, silver/copper wires?

Ears:

- Does the client have difficulty hearing you during the interview? Rough tests of hearing can be accomplished by ability to hear a whisper or rubbing fingers. Loss of hearing high-pitched sounds is common (presbycusis).
- Is there a buildup of cerumen in the ear or the presence of lesions?

Mouth/Nose:

- Does inspection reveal loose teeth or carries which can interfere with chewing and increase risk of infections and abscesses? Teeth may appear elongated as gums recede.
- Do the gums show evidence of gingivitis, red or white lesions (remove dentures if present). Atrophy of the gums is common after tooth loss.
- Does the tongue have any lesions or coating?
- Is there depappilation or a red beefy look that could indicate nutritional deficiencies?
- Does the client complain of dry mouth? This is common due to decreased saliva production. In the debilitated or NPO patient it can cause a thick mucous buildup in the absence of diligent mouth care.
- Do they complain of decreased taste? This is a common complaint and can effect nutritional status and is partially the result of decreased numbers of taste buds.

- Does the client complain of decreased smell? Smell is often diminished with aging and can further effect eating.

Neck:

- Is the neck normal on inspection and palpation?
- Can you palpate the thyroid? It is often hard to detect in the elderly.
- Is there evidence of adenopathy?

Inspection, Palpation and Auscultation of the Chest, Abdomen and Pelvis

Respiratory System:

- Is the chest normal on inspection?
- Is there decreased excursion?
- Are breath sounds significantly altered? This is not normal unless the client has disease. A decrease in respiratory efficiency is caused by decreased elasticity of the lung tissue, decreased number of alveoli and cilia, decreased secretions and decreased expendability of the chest due to increase in anteroposterior chest diameter and kyphosis.

Cardiovascular System:

- Does auscultation of the heart reveal murmurs or S_4 sounds common with aging?
- Decreased cardiac output in the elderly is the result of decreased elasticity of the heart and arteries. The heart is less able to generate a response to exercise, stress or increase fluid overloads.
- Are there premature beats? These are common, as are arrhythmias, although these are not normal with aging.
- Is there an increase in systolic and diastolic blood pressure? It is normal to see an increase up to 160/90 mm Hg. Postural hypotension is common due to decreased efficiency of the baroreceptors. This puts the older adult at increased risk of symptoms and falls as a result of medication or volume depletion.

- Is blood pressure hard to measure? While less common, calcification of the arteries can cause difficulty measuring the blood pressure because the arteries will not compress and relax with the cuff.
- Are pulses present and normal?

Abdomen, Rectum and Gastrointestinal System:

- Is the abdomen, pelvis and rectum appear normal to inspection and free of tenderness or masses?
- Is the abdomen protuberant? This is common with loss of muscle mass and tone.
- Are bowel sounds normal? Does the patient complain of constipation? Decreased peristalsis has been documented, but bowel sounds should not be decreased.
- Is liver size normal? While the liver is reported to be smaller in the older adult, this is not normally discernable on palpation.
- Does the rectum have normal sphincter tone? Is stool free of blood?

Kidneys and Urinary Tract:

- Do external organs appear normal to inspection?
- Does the client complain of frequent urination or nocturia? Bladder size decreases with age and there is decreased efficiency of bladder emptying which may result in findings of residual urine of 50-75cc.
- Does the client have incontinence? Incontinence is not normal with aging and should be evaluated for medical causes such as infection.
- The renal system is less efficient as a result of decreasd glomeruli, decreased blood flow and glomerular filtration rate. The result is decreased efficiency and can effect excretion of medication.

Reproductive System:

One of the most misunderstood concepts in the older adult is the need and desire to express one's sexuality. Despite common misconceptions, sexual function continues into at least the 8th decade of life, with potency in males and sexual interest in females. There have been few studies which have looked at sexuality in the older generation. Nevertheless, a healthy attitude toward intimacy and sexual expression should be encouraged.

Inclusive in the physical assessment should be questions regarding sexual activity, opening the discussion to feelings of anxiety and concern.

Rather than an intrusive question such as "Are you sexually active?," it may be more appropriate to ask, "Are there any difficulties with sexual function?" In this way, the client may respond without embarrassment. (Culturally, discussions of sexual activity were matters of privacy for this generation, in contrast to the norms of today's society.)

These questions can be included in the physical exam, when questioning normal and abnormal physical findings.

Female:

- Are the breasts free of lumps? The physical will reveal thinning of breast tissue in the older woman.

- Does the pelvic exam show atrophic vaginitis? This can result in painful intercourse and contribute to incontinence. These findings are the result of estrogen loss after menopause and may be altered in the female on estrogen replacement therapy. Thinning of pubic hair and presence of facial hair may also be the result of estrogen loss.

Male:

- Does exam reveal thinning of the pubic hair and decreased size of the testicles? These are common findings in the older male. Hernias are common.

- Is prostate enlarged?

Inspection and Examination of Neurological, Musculoskeletal System and Extremities:

Musculoskeletal Exam:

- Is there evidence of decreased muscle strength? While decreased tone and strength are common, they are not normal for aging and often the result of debilitation.

- Are there joint deformities or restrictions in range of motion? Findings of kyphosis, arthritis and osteoporosis are common.

Extremities and Feet:

- Do fingers show evidence of clubbing?

- Are feet free of findings? Inspect feet for general foot care, onchymycosis (fungal nails), calluses, bunions, toe deformities which might result in walking difficulty. Blisters or sores may suggest poor fitting shoes and can be serious in those with diabetes or vascular disease.

- Are other findings present on the extremities? Those related to cardiovascular system: venous stasis discoloration or decreased hair of the lower extremity. Pedal edema can signal congestive heart failure or signal more of a mechanical problem with poor venous return.

Neurological:

- Is there evidence of neurological deficits? Aging changes in the brain result in decreased numbers of neurons and decreased oxygenation, but should not effect physical functioning in the normal older adult.

- Testing of the cranial nerves should also be normal in the normal older adult. Occasionally decrease in upward gaze is seen in testing the Oculomotor nerve (III).

- Is there a tremor? Essential tremors are more likely to be familial, often occur in head and hands only, would not have other features of Parkinsonism such as cog-wheeling and flat facies.

- Is gait and balance normal?

- While most reflexes are normal in the elderly, ankle reflex is often absent and lower extremity reflexes may be slightly diminished.

- Is vibration sense decreased? This is a common finding in the elderly client.

Integumentary System

Skin:

- Are there observable changes? Normal changes result from a decrease in pigmentation, thinning of the dermis, slower healing, and a loss of the subcutaneous fat layer. Many of the visible aging changes result: graying of hair, wrinkles, pallor.

- Is there evidence of findings such as skin tags, seborrheic keratoses (flat brown oily), lentigines (liver spots), cherry hemangiomas (small red spots), actinic keratoses (flat lesions sometimes pale red or white on lips, often pre-cancerous)? Inspect to identify potentially cancerous lesions.

- Is the skin dry? Decreased sebaceous glands result in dry skin (xerosis) and diminished cooling response to heat through sweating.

Laboratory Findings

Laboratory studies are used to supplement the physical findings. In general, results of laboratory studies can vary widely among the elderly due to physiological changes, illness and medications. Age specific normals are not clear for most tests, but the majority of older adults could be expected to fall within the usual range of normal for most laboratory tests.

- Routine studies should be checked as part of a routine physical. A blood count, blood chemistries and urinalysis are recommended at least every two years for the older adult (unless otherwise indicated). Blood sugar should be checked yearly. Men may have a PSA (Prostate Screening Antigen) test every 1-2 years.

- Older adults may experience shifts in electrolytes even in minor illnesses and those with risk factors for alterations should be monitored routinely, such as clients taking diuretic medications.

- Cholesterol levels should be followed and steps taken to lower levels over 200 mg/dl. However, the risks vs. benefit of treatment for those with advanced age or at high risk for malnutrition should be evaluated.

- Older adults are at high risk for nutritional deficiencies. The appropriate daily allowances for the elderly are not known and their requirements may be higher than for the younger client. Evaluation of albumin (or pre-albumin) and protein should be done in the event of weight loss or poor nutrition. Deficiencies of Vitamin D, B_{12}, and calcium are common.

- Age can effect function of the endocrine glands and the efficiency of their feedback systems. Hypothyroidism is common and thyroid studies should be checked every two years.

PHYSICAL EXAMINATION FORM

Patient Name _____ Date _____

Record findings on physical examination and describe all abnormal findings/variations from normal.

<u>Vital Signs</u>

Weight _____ Height _____

BP supine _____ sitting _____ upright _____

P supine _____ sitting _____ upright _____

Orthostatic changes ____ Yes ____ No

<u>Head</u>

Temporal arteries _____ Normal _____

Abnormal (describe) _____

_____

Other (describe) _____

_____

Eyes

Able to read newsprint _____ With glasses _____ Without glasses
_____ Unable

| Acuity | Reading | R____/____ | L____/____ |
| | Distance | R____/____ | L____/____ |

Fields _____ Normal _____ Abnormal

Sclera/conjunctiva _____ Normal _____ Abnormal

Pupils _____ Normal _____ Iridectomy _____ R _____ L

Cataract _____ None _____ R _____ L

Fundi _____ Normal _____ Not seen _____ Abnormal

Describe abnormalities:_____

Ears

External canal _____ Normal _____ Cerumen

TMs _____ Normal _____ Not seen _____ Abnormal

Hearing _____ Hears normal voice _____ Impaired

_____ Wears aid _____ R _____ L

Describe abnormalities:_____

Nose

Septum/mucosa _____ Normal _____ Abnormal

Sinuses _____ Normal _____ Abnormal

Describe abnormalities:_____

Mouth

Lips _____ Nose _____ Cheilosis/angular stomatitis

Mucosa _____ Normal _____ Sores under dentures

_____ Other lesion(describe)

Tongue   _____ Normal   _____ Glossitis
                _____ Decreased papillation

Teeth   _____ Adequate for chewing _____ Poor hygiene
                _____ Edentulous _____ Dentures _____ Poor fit

Describe abnormalities: _____

_____

Neck

Thyroid   _____ Normal   _____ Abnormal (describe)

_____

_____

Lymphatic   No adenopathy   Abnormal (describe)
Cervical   _____   _____
Supraclavicular _____   _____
Axillary   _____   _____

_____

Breasts   _____ Masses   _____ None
                _____ Present (describe)

_____

_____

Lungs   Normal   Abnormal (describe)
Contour/Excursion _____   _____

_____

Breath Sounds   _____   _____

_____

Percussion   _____   _____

_____

Cardiovascular

Pulses

	Carotid	Radial	Femoral	Popliteal	DP	PT
R						
L						

Grade = 0, 1, 2

Bruits = B

Thrill = T

	Normal	Abnormal
Carotid Upstroke	_____	_____
Neck Veins	_____	_____
PMI	_____	_____
Rhythm	_____	_____
Heart Sounds	_____	_____ S3____S4

_____ Other (describe)

Murmur   _____ Absent   _____ Present

Rub   _____ Absent   _____ Present

Describe abnormalities:_____

Abdomen

Contour   _____ Normal   _____ Obese

                _____ Distended   _____ Other

Bowel sounds   _____ Normal   _____ Other

Bruits   _____ Absent   _____ Present

Tenderness   _____ Absent   _____ Present

Mass   _____Absent   _____Pulsatile_____Other

Liver span   _____cm

Spleen   _____Normal   _____Enlarged

Hernia   _____Absent   _____Present

Rectal   _____Normal   _____Other   _____Not done

Gualac   _____Negative _____Positive

Describe abnormalities: _____

<u>Genitourinary</u>   Normal   Abnormal (describe)

        _____   _____

_____

<u>Extremities</u>   Absent   Present

Clubbing/Cyanosis _____   _____

Edema   _____   _____

        _____ Pedal   _____ Tibial

Varicosities   _____   _____

Venous stasis   _____   _____   _____ Ulcers

Describe abnormalities: _____

_____

<u>Musculoskeletal</u>

Musculo-skeletal	Normal	Defor-mity	Limited ROM	Tender-ness	Inflam-mation
Back					
Neck					
Shoulder					
Wrists					
Hips					
Knees					
Other					

Describe: _____

Integumentary	Normal	Abnormal
Skin	_____	_____
Hair	_____	_____
Nails	_____	_____

Describe abnormalities:_____

_____

Cranial Nerves

Smell tested	_____ yes	_____ no
Able to detect	_____ yes	_____ no
Identifies smell	_____ yes	_____ no

	Normal	Abnormal
II	_____	_____
II,IV,VI	_____	_____
V	_____	_____
VII	_____	_____
VIII	_____	_____
IX	_____	_____
X	_____	_____
XI	_____	_____
XII	_____	_____

Describe abnormalities:_____

_____

Motor	Able	Unable
Stands on heels	_____	_____
Stands on toes	_____	_____
Touches top of head	_____	_____

	Absent	Present
Focal weakness	_____	_____
Proximal weakness	_____	_____
Atrophy	_____	_____
Spasticity	_____	_____
Cogwheeling	_____	_____
Bradykinesia	_____	_____
Tremor	_____ Resting	_____ Intention
Arm Drift	_____	_____

Describe abnormalities: _____

Sensory	Normal	Abnormal
Light touch	_____	_____
Vibratory	_____	_____
Pinprick	_____	_____
Proprioception	_____	_____

Reflexes

Primitives	_____ Absent	_____ Snout
		_____ Glabellar
		_____ Other

Describe abnormalities: _____

Reflexes

Describe abnormalities:

_____

_____

_____

_____

Describe abnormalities:

Cerebellar	Normal	Abnormal
FTN	_____	_____
HKS	_____	_____

Romberg	Able eyes open	Able eyes closed
feet together	_____	_____
semi-tandem	_____	_____
tandem	_____	_____

	Able	Unable
neck rotation	_____	_____
neck extension	_____	_____
trunk flexion	_____	_____

Describe abnormalities:_____
_____

Gait

With_____without_____assistive device

Short steps _____ Shuffle _____ Lack arm swing _____

Flexed/stooped posture _____ Turns en bloc _____

Wide-based _____ Poor tandem _____ Other _____

Steps/12 ft_____ Steps for turn_____

Describe abnormalities:_____
_____

Interpretation: Record all abnormal findings to identify problems for evaluation. The physical examination should be combined with the history, psychosocial, functional and cognitive assessment. Identify problems for referral.

Nursing Implications:

Findings from the Physical Examination will be used give further information for identifying medical problems and treatments indicated. This will assist the nurse in providing the client with:

- Information regarding medical problems, the etiology, prognosis and anticipated progression

- Education regarding medications or treatments, identifying potential complications and preventive measures. For example, teaching the client with peripheral vascular disease or diabetes regarding good foot care to prevent infection

- Referral to community resources for information or assistance in managing medical problems such as the local Heart Association, Cancer Society, or other organizations

- Recommendation of appropriate follow-up to monitor ongoing problems.

CASE STUDY

Mrs. Jones is a 77 year old black widow who comes to the nurse-managed clinic complaining of fatigue and nurse Thompson is assigned to complete the assessment.

History:

Mrs. Jones has been relatively healthy all of her life. She has been treated for high blood pressure for the past five years with a diuretic medication, hydrochlorothiazide. She could tell the reason for the medication, its name and how to take it appropriately. Mrs. Jones says she feels tired all of the time, and some days just doesn't want to do anything, even getting dressed. The fatigue is worse some days, but doesn't seem related to any particular activity. Mrs. Jones complains of feeling cold a lot of the time. She has lost ten pounds over the past six months.

Functional Assessment:

Mrs. Jones is independent in all of her basic Activities of Daily Living. Her only problem is with mobility. She walks with a cane and has difficulty going up and down stairs. She has fallen twice in the last month. Once she fell on the way to the bathroom in the middle of the night. A second fall occurred when she got up from her sofa to go answer the telephone. She is fearful of falling again.

Mrs. Jones daughter is assisting with many of her Instrumental Activities of Daily Living. She does most of the grocery shopping, although Mrs. Jones usually gives her a list and money for the purchases. Sometimes Mrs. Jones goes with her and will participate in the shopping, picking out and paying for groceries. The daughter helps with heavy housework and laundry and will have her mother over for meals once or twice each week. Mrs. Jones does all the daily cleaning, dishes and making her bed. She pays her own bills. Mrs. Jones cooks for herself. Recently she has not been fixing complete meals as much as she used to because of the fatigue. She does not drive or have a car and takes the bus to church, to the clinic, to visit her sister or to the store. Recently, she will only go places when the daughter takes her, partly because of her fatigue and her fear of falling. She calls the daughter or sons when she needs any assistance.

Psychosocial Assessment:

Mrs. Jones has been a widow for 12 years, and has three children. Her single daughter lives upstairs in the two-family flat that they own. Her two sons are married and have children and live nearby. Mrs. Jones has an older sister in a nursing home. The daughter can assist her anytime she needs any help, but the daughter works full-time during the week. Mrs. Jones used to be fairly involved with her church, would visit the sister twice each week and go the senior center once a week. Mrs. Jones income is adequate to meet her needs. Mrs Jones has no history of mental illness or depression, although she says she feels down a lot more than usual lately. Her score on the Geriatric Depression Scale is 5. Mrs. Jones would score as having Good Social Relationships on the OARS Social Resource Scale; however, if the recent decline in her activities and getting out would continue, she would move to the level of Mildly Socially Impaired, due to decline in social relationships. Her daughter could take care of her indefinitely, if necessary.

Cognitive Assessment:

Mrs. Jones scores 6 on the Short Blessed Test for cognitive impairment. She does not seem to have any memory impairment, and probably did as poorly as she did on the test because she has only a 5th grade education, (this usually effects test performance). She would be considered within the normal range.

Positive Findings on Physical Assessment:

Mrs. Jones blood pressure is 120 /60. She experiences a drop of 20 mm Hg systolic and 10 mm Hg diastolic blood pressure upon arising from lying to standing, and feels wobbly. Mrs. Jones has some trouble with vision, even with her glasses and a cataract in her right eye. She has some premature beats on auscultation of the heart. Lower extremities are weak and she has arthritis of the right knee which gives her some pain. She has a cane she bought at the drug store, but it is too tall for her height. Mrs. Jones has dry, flaky skin on her legs and arms, and corns and calluses on her feet.

Abnormal Laboratory Findings:

Mrs. Jones has a low thyroid level, and low potassium. Her albumin is at the low end of the normal range, other tests are normal.

Findings:

Mrs. Jones is beginning to experience problems and the first signs of frailty as her function declines. Intervention now can prevent her from developing complications of her medical problems or poor nutrition, injury as a result of her physical frailty and depression and isolation. The following problems and recommendations are designed to keep Mrs. Jones active and productive for as long as possible.

Care Plan:

<u>Problems -- Discussion/Recommendations</u> -- History of hypertension: Mrs. Jones blood pressure is not very high at this time, and she is experiencing postural hypotension. She may no longer need treatment for her hypertension, and can avoid the risk of falls and hypokalemia if she can do without the diuretic.

Hypokalemia: Potassium replacement may be indicated, and the hypokalemia may be contributing to her fatigue. Instruction on a high potassium diet may be needed if she continues to take the diuretic medication.

Hypothyroidism: Thyroid replacement may improve her fatigue, dry skin and feeling cold easily. Her blood levels should be monitored every 3-6 months.

<u>Potential for Alteration in Nutrition</u>

Mrs. Jones is at risk for nutritional deficiency if her diet in nutrition does not improve. Many older adults who live alone are bored with cooking and eating. She could be referred to Meals On Wheels for some lunches through the week. A schedule of several meals each week with her daughter would provide some socialization, as would attending the lunch program at the senior center. She could take a multiple vitamin with minerals to supplement her diet.

Potential for Injury

Mrs. Jones has several risk factors for falls. She has poor vision, needing new glasses and should see an eye doctor to evaluate her cataract. Another risk factor is her arthritis, cane and lower extremity weakness. She would benefit from a regular exercise program for muscle strengthening, a cane that is fit specifically for her and a check to make sure she uses it correctly. The cane would also help take the stress off her arthritic knee to help prevent inflammation and pain. She would also benefit from good foot care to treat her corns and calluses, and should wear supportive shoes (such as athletic or walking shoes) that fit well. Mrs. Jones also has some postural hypotension. She could do some leg exercises before arising, flexing and extending her feet a few times. She should also be instructed to get up slowly, and to use her cane when arising. Place grab bars around the toilet, so that she has something to hold onto when she goes to the bathroom at night. Mrs. Jones had some premature heart beats which seem nonsignificant, but if she continues to fall with no reason, a cardiac evaluation would be indicated.

Potential for Social Isolation

Mrs. Jones may return to her normal activities with treatment of the above problems, which will increase her socialization and probably improve her mood. She might benefit in the future from information about community resources that would allow her to continue activities if she has trouble using the public transportation, or getting to her senior center. Many cities provide special transportation services for older adults. Some programs such as adult day care provide their own transportation and some additional support for people with more disability. Adult day care also provides socialization, meals and some supervision, if needed.

References

The forms and assessment procedures were adapted from the Program on Aging Geriatric Assessment Center, Washington University, St. Louis, Missouri

Functional Assessment

Katz, S., Ford, A.B., Moskowitz, R.S., Jackson, B.A., & Jaffe, M.W. "Studies of illness in the aged. The index of ADL: A standardized measure of physiological and psychosocial function". *JAMA*, 185:94-98, (1963).

Granger, C.V. et al. "Outcome of comprehensive medical rehabilitation: Measure of PULSES profile and the Barthel index". *Archives of Physical and Medical Rehabilitation*, 60:145-154, (1979).

Lawton, M.P. "The functional assessment of elderly people". *Journal of the American Geriatrics Society*, 19(6, 465-481, (1971).

Lawton, H.P., and Brody, E.M. *Assessment of older people: Self-maintaining and instrumental activities of daily living.* Gerontologist 9:179, (1969).

Mahoney, R.I., & Barthel, D.W. "Functional evaluation: The Barthel Index". *Maryland State Medical Journal* 14:61-65, (1965).

Pfeiffer, E. (Ed.). *Multidimensional function assessment: The OARS Methodology.* 2nd Edition. Durham NC: Duke University Press, (1978).

Mental Status Tests

Katzman, R. et al, "Validation of a short orientation memory-concentration test of cognitive impairment". *American Journal of Psychiatry*, 140:734-739, (1983).

Folstein, M.E., Folstein, S.E. & McHugh, P.R. "Mini-mental state: A practical method for grading the cognitive state of patients for the clinician." *Journal of Psychiatric Research* 12:189-198, (1975).

Pfeiffer, E. "A short portable mental status questionnaire for the assessment of organic brain deficit in elderly patients". *Journal of the American Geriatrics Society*, 23:433-441, (1975).

Depression Screening

Beck, A.T., & Beck, R.W. "Screening depressed patients in family practice: A rapid technique". *Postgraduate Medicine:*52(6) 81-85, (1972).

Hamilton, M. "A rating scale for depression". *J Neurolo Neurosurg Psychiatry* 23:56-62, (1960).

Hays, A.M., & Borger, F. "A test in time". *AJN*, 85 (10):1107-1111, (1985).

Zung, W.K. "A self rating depression scale". *Archives of General Psychiatry.* 12(1) 63-70, (1965).

Assessment References

Anderson, G.P. "A fresh look at assessing the elderly". RN, June 28-40, (1989).

Bruggraf, V., & Donlon, B. "Assessing the elderly system by system". *AJN*, 974-984. (1985).

Gallo, J.J., Reichel, W., & Anderson, L. *Handbook of geriatric assessment.* Rockville, MN: Aspen Publishers, (1988).

Henderson, M.L. "Altered presentations". *AJN*, 85 (10):1104-1106 (1985).

Kane, R.A., & Kane, R.L. *Assessing the elderly: A practical guide to measurement.* MA: Lexington Books (1981).

Leukenotte, A.G. *Gerontological Assessment.* St. Louis: CV Mosby, (1991).

General References

American Psychiatric Association. *Diagnostic and Statistical Manual of Mental Disorders* (4th ed.), Washington, D.C.: American Psychiatric Press (1994).

Beck, A.T. and Emery, G. *Anxiety and Phobias: A Cognitive Perspective.* New York: Basic Books (1985)

Blazer, D.G. *Depression in Late Life.* St. Louis, MO: C.V. Mosby. (1982)

Blow, F. "Screening for substance abuse among the elderly". Paper presented at the 7th Annual Meeting of the American Association for Geriatric Psychiatry, New Orleans, LA. February 13, 1993.

Buchsbaum, D.G., Buchanan, R.G., Welsh, J., Centor, R.M., and Schnoll, S.H. "Screening for Drinking Disorders in the Elderly Using the CAGE Questionnaire". *Journal of the American Geriatric Society* 40:622-665 (1992)

Eberale, P. and Hess, P. *Towards Health Aging.* St. Louis, MO: The C.V. Mosby (1981)

Erikson, E.H. "The Human Life Cycle". In D.L. Sills (ed.), *International Encyclopedia of the Social Sciences.* New York: MacMillan 268-292. (1968)

Folstein, M.F., Folstein, S.E. and McHugh, P.R. "Mini Mental State: A Practical Methods for grading the Cognitive State of Patients for the American". *Journal of Psychiatric Research,* 12:189-198 (1975)

Grossberg, G.T., Manepalli, J., and Solomon, K. "Diagnosis of Depression in Demented Patients". In J.E. Morley, R. Strong, R. Coe, and G.T. Grossberg (eds.), *Memory Function and Aging Related Disorders.* New York: Springer, 237-247 (1992)

Hall, G. and Buckwalter, K. "Progressively Lowered Stress Threshold: A Conceptualized Model for Care of Adults with Alzheimer's Disease". *Archives of Psychiatric Nursing* 1(1), 399-406 (1987).

Hackinski, V., Iliff, L., Zilhka, E., et al "Cerbreal Blood Flow in Dementia". *Archives of Neurology* 32:632-637 (1975).

Havinghurst, R. J. *Developmental Tasks and Education.* New York: David McKay (1972).

Holman, A. *Family Assessment: Tools for Understanding and Intervention.* Beverly Hills:Sage (1983).

Kermis, M. *Mental Health in Late Life and Adaptive Process.* Boston:Jones and Bartlett Publications (1986)

Mace, N.L. "The Management of Problem Behaviors". in N. Moore (ed.), *Dementia Care Patient, Family and Community.* Baltimore, MD:Johns Hopkins University Press, 74-112 (1990).

Mace, N.L. and Rabins, P.V. *The 36-Hour Day.* Baltimore:Johns Hopkins University Press (1981).

Maslow A. *The S-I test: A measure of psychological security-insecurity.* Stanford, CA:Stanford University Press.

Mayfield, D., McCleod, G., Hall, P. "The CAGE Questionnaire: Validation of a new alcoholism screening instrument". *American Journals of Psychiatry* 131:1121 (1974).

McGoldrick, M., and Gerson, R. *Genograms in Family Assessment.* New York: W.W. Norton (1985)

Peck, R.C. "Psychological Developments in the Second Half of Life". In B.L. Neugarten (ed.), *Middle Age and Aging*, Chicago, University of Chicago Press.(1986)

Pfieffer, E. "A short portable mental status questionnaire for the assessment of organic brain deficit in elderly patients". *Journal of American Geriatric Society* 23:433-437 (1975).

Reisberg, B. *Alzheimer's Disease.* New York:The Free Press (1983)

Sharpiro, S., Skinner, E., Kessler, L. et al "Utilization of health and mental health services: Three epidemiologic catchment area sites". *Archives of General Psychiatry* 41:971 (1984).

Shamoian, C.A. "Somatic Therapies in Geriatric Psychiatry", In L.W. Lazarris (ed.), *Essentials of Geriatric Psychiatry.* New York:Springer Publishing Co. 173-189.

Sparacino, J. "Industrial Psychotherapy with the Aged: A Selective Review". *International: Journal of Aging and Human Development* 9, 197-220.

Szwabo P.A. and Boesch, K. "Impact of Personality and Personality Disorders in the Elderly". In P.A. Szwabo and G.T. Grossberg (eds.) *Problem behavior in Long Term Care Recognition Diagnosis and Treatment*. New York:Springer 237-247 (1993).

Yesavage, J.A. and Brink, T.L. "Development and Validation of a Geriatric Screening Scale: A Preliminary Report". *Journal of Psychiatric Research,* 17(1), 37-49 (1983).

Zarit, S., Zarit, S. "Depression in later life: Theory and Assessment". In Abrahams J.P., Crooks, V.S. (eds.) *Geriatric Mental Health*. New York, Grune and Stratton. (1984).

Unit 1 - Chapter 4

Mental Health Of The Elderly

Mentally healthy aging has many definitions and concepts Many concepts of normal are sterotypical in nature. The same notion of physical and mental health should be applied to any age. A mentally healthy person gives evidence of:

    Positive self attitude

    Growth and self-actualization

    Reality perception

    Integration of personality

    Autonomy

    Environmental mastery

The goal of mental health intervention is to assist in maximizing potential abilities and resources. Stressful events, i.e. death of a spouse, child, pet, onset of illness, financial insecurity, trigger new and chronic psychiatric symptoms. These trigger events are related to:

    1. Lack of control over situations and environment

    2.. Fears of dependency

    3. Feelings of helplessness

I. Developmental Tasks of Aging Theories

A. Erikson (1968): Ego Integrity vs. Despair

If one cannot accept that life has been meaningful, appropriate and worthwhile, there is depression, bitterness, anger and fear of death.

B. Peck (1968): Ego differentiation vs. Work preoccupation

When work role is lost, individuals need to redefine and reappraise their personal world.

<u>Body Transcendence vs. Body preoccupation</u>
Adaptation to change in bodily function or become preoccupied with their bodies.

<u>Ego Transcendence vs. Ego preoccupation</u>
Active process to gain closure on one's life, a period of re-evaluation of past, dealing with present and the future

C. Havighurst (1972): Developmental Tasks of Late Life

1. Adjusting to declining physical strength and health
2. Adjusting to retirement and its reduced income
3. Adjusting to changes in the health of one's spouse
4. Establishing an explicit affiliation with one's age group.
5. Adopting and adapting social roles in flexible way.
6. Establishing satisfactory physical living arrangements.

II. Loss

With increasing age, older adults experience a variety of physical, social and psychological losses. These losses may affect mobility and environment increasing the risk of isolation. The focus of the developmentalists is that aging presents a great adaptive challenge. If met with flexibility, there is adaptation; if met with inflexibility, there is maladaptation. Coping mechanisms are developed throught the person's lifetime and likewise can facilitate the adjustment to stress and loss.

A. Assessment of loss; Major issues

Impact of disease and diagnosis upon current level of functioning.

1. Assess client's understanding of illness, treatment, prognosis, and management.

2. Effects of disease, symptoms, diagnosis, life-style, mobility, self-care capacity (IADL, ADL)

3. Reactions to illness and fears of suffering, dying and death; body image

4. Identify cognitive beliefs about illness both accurate and perceived

B. Physiologic response to loss

Evaluation of psychological or mental status changes, includes a thorough history and physical.

1. In older adults, confusion or mental status symbols may be the first sign of a physical problem or illness.

2. A medical history assesses overall functioning, capabilities and identification of current and potential problems.

3. Evaluation of medications is essential, noting dosage and compliance, use of over the counter preparations and vitamins, and frequency of use.

   - The elderly regularly use pain relievers, laxatives, vitamins and sleeping aids. Other remedies and herbal preparations need to be identified since these have similar properties as prescribed drugs.

4. Use of alcohol and illicit drugs, i.e. marijuana, cocaine, needs ot be assessed. Related questions;

   a. What do you drink, how much, how often?

   b. Previous treatment for alcohol problems?

   c. Family history of alcohol abuse

   d. Useful tools are the CAGE (Buchanan, Buschbaum, Welsch, et al., 1992) and MAST-G (Blow, 1993)

III. Psychosocial Examination

A. Social Support
1. Who is important to the client and current relationships?
2. Health and or loss of health.
3. Satus of spouse, sibling, friends, neighbors
4. Knowledge of community resources and other agencies
5. Use of ECOMAP (Holman, 1983) and Genogram (Mcgoldrick and Ferson, 1985) may be helpful
   - A way of diagramming the resources and connections between the individual, family, resources and other individuals involved.
   - Provides a picture of demands and resources of the individual/family system.
   - Genograms are tools which assess for the learning about the family's history and relationships over time.

B. Social Role
1. Adjustment from work role to retirement identity
2. Role changes in the couple and in the family
3. Adjustments to retirement and leisure time
4. Counseling needs
5. Referral to community resources

C. Socialization
1. Has stress and illness affected activities, involvement and opportunity?
2. How is time spend and is the individual satisfied with life?
3. As related, are there finances and transportation available to access activities?

D. Economics
1. Loss of income; adjusting to fixed income
2. Losses of previously enjoyed life style and pursuits

3. Ability to afford health care insurance, meds

4. Adequate housing or issues in leaving one's home for other older adult alternatives

E. Cognition

Cognitive appraisal and assessment is important when deterioration of memory and intellectual funcitoning is suspected. Since the incidence of dementia is significant in the elderly, several screening tools are available to assess memory and function. The brief tests determine orientation for person, place, time, recent and remote memory and calculations such as the Short Protable Mental Status Questionnaire (SPMSQ).

Other intstruments tap higher levels of functioning by asking questions to check abstract thinking and simple problems solving such as the Folstein Mini Mental Status Examination (MMSE,1975). The MMSE is the cognitive test recommended by the National Institute of Neurological and Communication Disorders and Stroke, as well as the Alzheimer's Disease and Related Disorders Association. Caution about the use of these tools:

1. Screening tools, supplemental information and diagnostic work up are essential in ruling out other treatable conditons.

2. Caution is advised to avoid prematurely eliminating the client as a source of information if incorrect answers on testing occurs. Clients with spotty recognition abilities may be capable of answering questions about activities, relationships, moods or preferences.

3. Language or cultural barriers may create an obstacle in administering the tests

4. Disease, neurologic dysfunction or learning disorders may affect ability to follow directions within the testing framework.

IV. Psychiatric Disorders of the Elderly

The eldery have a higher incidence of psychopathology than other age groups. After age 65, it is estamated that 50 percent of this population will experience psychiatric symptoms or pathology. With age, there is a greater risk for progressive deteriorating dementias, and higher rates of and under diagnosed depression. Increasing physical illnesses, chronicity and subsequent physical limitations further increase their risks of psychiatric symptoms and disorders.

A. The Geriatric Psychiatric Assessment

1. Goal of psychiatric assessment is to gather and intergrate biologic, psychologic and socioeconomic data to provide comprehensive understanding of a person's psychosocial status.

    a. Identify previously identified medical and psychiatric diagnoses

    b. Identify psychosocial evaluation to gather information on past coping abilities

    c. Assess stressors and resources

    d. Assess factors to enhance or inhibit treatment

    e. Evaluate individual's developmental disabilities

    f. Explore work/education history

    g. Assess marital/relationship history

    h. Examine resources: including housing, finances

2. Psychodynamic assessment attempts to evaluate some unconscious or interpersonal motivation for a person's behavior in attempt to understand this behavior.

3. Needs assessment (Maslow's Hierarchy of Needs, 1952) identifies basic issues such as feelings of love, self-esteem, interpersonal needs and self-actualization

4. Mental Status Examination

    MSE delineates psychopathological symptoms to ensure accurate/appropriate assessment of psychosocial status of older clients. Includes;

    a. Appearance

    b. Level of consciousness/alertness

    c. Attention span

    d. Mood

    e. Affect

    f. Activity level

    g. Speech

    h. Thought process

    i. Content of thought

    j. Perception

    k. Memory

    l. Orientation

    m. Intelligence

    n. Judgement

    o. Insight

5. Treatment planning/conference

    - Discussion and synthesis of information with the treatment team, client and family and development of a plan of action.

B. Major Affective Disorders (MAD)

Most common among the elderly and are highly treatable disorders. MAD significantly intereferes with quality of life and life functions. Fifteen percent of general populations over 65 years of age experience symptoms of depression.

1. Prevalence of Mood Disorders
   a. 12% - 15% of population over 76 yrs. of age
   b. 15% - 20% of nursing home residents
   c. Third most frequent psychiatric disorders in extended care facilities
   d. 30% of individuals with dementia have depression
2. Symptoms of depression
   a. Depressed mood
   b. Loss of interest or plesure
   c. Weight loss
   d. Appetite changes
   e. Sleep disturbance
   f. Psychomotor agitation or retardation
   g. Decreased energy or fatigue
   h. Feelings of worthlessness or guilt
   i. Decreased concentration
   j. Recurrent thoughts of death or suicide
      *** 5 of 9 must be present day to day for at least two weeks to constitute diagnosis of 'major depression.'
3. Geriatric Presentation of Depression
   a. Masked-Client denies any 'depression' or mood changes, despite effects on appetite, activities and enjoyment
   b. Somatic-Client voices depression through vague physical complaints that are unfounded in physical exam and medical work-up
   c. Life-Review-Client is preoccupied with past events in an attempt to resolve it, or is depressed and distraught with life outcomes.

4. Pseudomentia-A depression that mimics the cognitive impairment of dementia
5. Dysthymia
   - Occurs in 2% of mood disorders; diagnosed when depression mood is present most of the time for at least 2 years with no remissions longer than 2 months and at least 2 of the following symptoms;
   a. Poor appetite or overeating
   b. Sleep changes
   c. Fatigue
   d. Low self-esteem
   e. Poor concentration or difficulty making decisions
   f. Feelings of hopelessness
6. Bipolar disorder
   - Occurs in 10% of cases. Geriatric presentation;
   a. Elderly are more likely to be irritable than euphoric
   b. Dysphoria, confusion, cognitive changes and impairment of concentration and attention may be present
   c. Generally occurs during 30's and 40's but recurrent episodes of mania and/or depression continue into old age
   d. Occasionally episodes can occur for first time in late life
   e. Symptoms include;
      - Overactivity
      - Pressure of speech, e.g. talking too much, too fast
   f. Distractability
   g. Decreased sleep
   h. Overspending
   i. Hoarding
   j. Grandiosity

k. Mood may be elevated, irritable or labile

* Requires at least three of these symptoms for diagnosis.

**These signs and symptoms are typical of manic phase. If not actually seen by physician, may be diagnosed as dysthymia.

C. Medical Evaluation of Depression
   1. Look for psychosocial triggers
   2. Look for drug toxicity
   3. Look for underlying medical problems
   4. Perform neuro-psychiatric and physical evaluation
   5. Evaluate labs; CBC, UA, Chem 18, RPR, HIV, TSH, B12, RBC, Folate and CXR, EKG
   6. Assessment should inlcude;
      a. Changes in physical, psychological functioning
      b. Functional changes in ADI /IADL
      c. Evaluation of anti-depressants
         - For atypical depressive or non-responders, consider a monamine oxidase inhibitor (MAOI), e.g., Parnate, Nardil or Marplan
      d. Appropriateness of ECT therapy, especially in psychotic or delusional cases

D. Anti-depressant Therapy
   1. Recommendations for ECT
      a. Individuals who are suicidal or homicidal
      b. Resistant depression
      c. Intolerance of antidepressant side effects
      d. Malignant hypertension
      e. Emergency or life-threatening situation (suicidal)
      f. Previous success with ECT

g. Anti-depressant therapy more effective post ECT

2. Rules of Anti-depressant Treatment Summary

   a. Pick drug with best profile, i.e., low anticholinergic and cardiac side effects

   b. Give small test dose and increase gradually 'Start low, go slow.'

   c. Maintain at therapeutic dose for 4-8 weeks

   d. Treat acute episode for 9-12 mos.; consider long term maintenance at therapeutic dose to prevent relapse

   e. Routine blood levels of drug as well as CBC, SMA6,

   f. Monitor for adverse effects

   g. Quantify measurements of change through administration of Geriatric Depression Scale

E. Suicide

1. 70-74 yr. old caucasian males have the highest rate of suicide in the United States

2. Risk factors include;

   a. Living alone

   b. Depression

   c. Chronic or acute illness

   d. Recent (1 mo.) physican office visit

3. Highest risk includes;

   a. Previous suicide attempts

   b. Suicide plan

   c. Family history of suicide

4. Assessment includes these two questions;

   a. "Have you ever felt so bad you thought you'd like to kill yourself?"

b. "What would you do?"
5. Refer to psychiatrist, mental health facility, mental health specialists or family physician

F. Treatment of major depression includes any combination of the following;
1. Psychotherapeutic/Behavioral
2. Supportive or dynamic therapy; individual and group
3. Biofeedback/relaxation therapy
4. Cognitive therapy
5. Biologic therapies
6. Bright light therapy
7. Sleep deprivation
8. Tricyclic anti-depressants
9. MAO inhibitors
10. Second generation anti-depressants
11. Selective serotonin reuptake inhibitors (SSRI's)
12. Electroconvulsive Therapy (ECT)

G. Anti-Depressant Therapy
1. Choice of a secondary amine, e.g., Nortriptyline or Desipramine may be a drug of choice in 'younger and healthier' elderly.
2. Be aware of anticholinergic effects
3. Mild sedation
4. Orthostasis
5. Cardiac toxicity

6. In 'older and frail' elderly;
   a. Selective serotonin reuptake inhibitors (SSRI's), e.g., sertraline (Zoloft), paroxetine (Paxil), and fluoxetine (Prozac) or Buproprion (Wellbutrin) are drugs of choice.

V. Anxiety

A. Definition includes;
   1. Unrealistic, excessive anxiety, worry about two or more life circumstances for at least 6 months
   2. Symptoms occur more often than not
   3. Does not occur as a symptom of another disorder such as depression
   4. If another disorder is present, the focus or symptoms are unrelated to that disorder; i.e. worry about having an attack in panic disorders

B. Symptoms and complaints include;
   1. Tremor, trembling, shakiness
   2. Muscle tension, aches
   3. Fatigability
   4. Restlessness
   5. Smothering feelings, shortness of breath
   6. Dry mouth, sweating
   7. Nausea, diarrhea, gastrointestinal distress
   8. Flashes or flushes
   9. Frequent urination
   10. Swallowing difficulties
   11. Dizziness
   12. Feeling edgy, nervous

13. Concentration difficulties
14. Sleep difficulties
15. Palpitations
16. Irritability
17. Startle response
18. Clammy hands

C. Diagnostic tests to rule out other medical problems;
1. Cardiovascular
2. Respiratory
3. Parkinson's Disease
4. Movement disorder
5. Thyroid disease

D. Assessment includes;
1. Personality style and/or disorder
2. Polypharmacy
3. Substance abuse
4. Drug withdrawl
5. Environmental changes or stress
6. Social network and resources

E. Treatment goals;
1. Eliminate excessive disability
2. Stabilize present coping abilities
3. Change behavior and/or coping strategies
4. Support

F. Treatment approaches;
1. Behavioral therapy including biofeedback, progressive muscle relaxation, guided imagery

2. Cognitive behavioral therapy

3. Psychotherapies including milieu

4. Family therapy and support

5. Medications;

   a. Short half-life anxiolytics, Buspirone, Alprazolam,etc. Serotonin reuptake inhibitors have been effective particularly in panic disorders i.e., Sertraline, Paroxetine

VI. Personality Styles and Disorders

A. Defined as an individual's life long style of interacting with people and the environment. Personality style of behaving does not necessarily interfere with daily functioning or with interaction.

1. Personality styles include;

   a. Dependent

   b. Clinging

   c. Indecisive

   d. Stubborness

   e. Feisty

   f. Controlling

   g. Manipulative

   h. Irritable

2. Personality disorders;

   a. Passive aggressive

   b. Passive dependent

   c. Obsessive-compulsive

   d. Paranoid

B. Personality disorder characteristics
    1. Maladaptive interactional patterns with family, friends, etc.
    2. Heavy focus on somatic concerns
    3. Depressive withdrawl
    4. High incidence of comorbidity of depression
    5. Assessment includes;
        a. Episodic or chronic behaviors
        b. Is this a life long or a new behavior ?
        c. Does the behavior interfere with daily functioning?
C. Obsessive Compulsive personality characteristics
    1. Perfectionistic
    2. Inflexible
    3. Unable to express warm feelings
    4. Preoccupied with detail
    5. Dislikes changes
D. Passive Dependent personality characteristics
    1. Relies on others
    2. Lacks adequate skills to deal effectively with others
    3. Dependency needs met by others
E. Paranoid personality characteristics
    1. Suspicious
    2. Cautious
    3. Wary of others' motives
    4. Mistrust of others
    5. Unwilling to share emotions
    6. Constant sense of shame and humiliation

F. Passive Agressive personality characteristics
   1. Passively resists requests to perform
   2. Indirectly resents and opposes demands by use of procrastination, dawdling
   3. Forgetfulness and inefficiency
   4. Fails to do their part or share of activity
   5. Can be sulky, argumentative
   6. Irritable
   7. Critical and scornful
G. Treatment of personality disorders
   1. Treat primary diagnosis first, e.g. depression
   2. Create effective relationship with interdisciplinary treatment team and family in defining treatment plan
   3. Set clean, realistic goals for both use of psycho-therapies and somatic therapies based on holistic assessment of individual's long term functioning
   4. Focus on present reality and relationships
H. Treatment concerns
   1. Elderly individuals with personality disorders in old age are ill equipped to cope with its stressors.
   2. Elderly individuals experience loss as more narcissistic assaults and respond by increasing manipulation of care providers, often resulting in a good guy-bad buy split.
   3. Elderly individuals have difficulty grieving and intolerance of anxiety symptoms which make these individuals a treatment challenge.

VII. Schizophrenia, Paraphrenia and Paranoid Disorders

A. Schizophrenia

1. Rarely occurs for first time in old age

2. Occurrence in old age is usually termed paraphrenia, affecting 1.5% of the elderly population

3. Compartmentalized paranoid delusions more commonly seen

4. Functioning (IADL/ADL) may not be effected

5. Treatment: psychosocial and environmental, mileu, using the environment of structure, safety and support as part of the treatment

6. Antipsychotics may not be necessary if ADL's and usual functioning are not affected

B. Schizophrenia, Chronic

1. Persists into old age

2. Symptoms include disturbances in;

    a. Behavior

    b. Affect

    c. Thought

    d. Activity

    e. Perception

3. Presentation includes;

    a. Acute psychosis diminishes in aging

    b. Symptoms may be burned out

    c. May be isolated, have little or no family involved, or estranged from loved ones

4. Assessment includes;

    a. Need for antipsychotics (may need lesser dose)

    b. Social support

    c. Community resources including case management services to insure adequate health/psychiatric care, housing and finances

5. Treatment concerns;

    a. Tardive Dyskinesia (TD) in long term use of psychotropics

       • TD is an extrapyramidal disorder associated with the use of antipsychotic drugs. Symptoms usually present as buccal lingual facial movement, e.g. puckering, licking, sucking, chewing, and swallowing movement. Can be involuntary tongue and facial movements.

    b. Abnormal involuntary movements of neck, legs, chest, arms, bladder dynsfunction

B. Paranoia

1. Defined by delusions-fixed unshakable beliefs

2. Symptoms can include;

    a. Suspiciousness

    b. Mistrust

    c. Isolation

    d. Eccentricity

    e. Acting on unfounded beliefs

    f. Anxiety

    g. Anger, resentment and violence

3. Need to assess;

    a. Sensory deficits and auditory changes

       • Noted increased incidence of hearing loss with suspiciousness

b. Medication/ ETOH use, review for side effects

   c. Isolation-deteriorating/changing neighborhood

   d. Relocation-a recent move

4. Determine;

   a. Whether symptoms are based in reality

   b. Degree of intensity

      - Are delusions relatively compartmentalized or encompassing one's life and interfering with daily functions?

5. Psychosocial interventions;

   a. Supportive and clear communication

   b. Trust and empathetic understanding

   c. Community resources

   d. Safe environment

   e. Treat anxiety with behavioral approaches and/or symptom relieving medication

   f. Reduce environmental threat with alternative explanations of what is happening to them

VIII. Progressive Deteriorating Dementia

A. Incidence

   1. Senile Dementia of Alzheimer's Type (SDAT) 52%

   2. Multi-Infarct Dementia -- 17%

   3. Mixed -- 14%

   4. Other -- 15%

B. Types;

   1. Familial; Chromosome 14 and 19

   2. Non-familial; Occurence of disease is random and is not associated with higher family incidence

C. Epidemiology of Dementia
    1. 4 million Americans
    2. 50% of nursing home residents
    3. Incidence is greater as one ages;
        - Approximately 40% of the age of 85
D. Etiology-Current theories
    1. Reversible causes;
        a. Electrolyte or metabolic imbalance; dehydration
        b. Lyme disease; early recognition and treatment
        c. Drug toxicity
        d. Inflammatory disease
        e. Syphilis; tertiary not reversible
        f. Alcohol symdrome
        g. Nutritional deficits
    2. Irreversible causes
        a. Vascular disease
        b. Slow virus
        c. Toxins
        d. Defective immune system
        e. Neurotransmitter depletion
E. Neurochemical changes
    1. Cortical neuron loss
    2. Loss of dendrites
        - The dendrite of the neuron makes up the primary surface for reception and interaction with other neurons. Loss of dendrites plus neuron reduction and shrinkage affect nerve cell numbers and the neuro-chemical interaction and transmissions.

3. Neuronal atrophy
   - Degenerative (shrinkage) of neurons which makes the neurochemical transmissions ineffective
4. Neuroanatomic change-found on autopsy
   - Neurofibrillary tangles
   - Neurotic plaques

F. Differential Diagnosis
   1. Evaluation of delirium;
      - Rule out and treat possible causes of cognitive impairment i.e., infection, injury, trauma and medication
   2. Diagnosis of dementia;
      - Insure a dementia workup is completed
   3. Dementia vs. depression;
      a. Depression is defined as feelings of sadness, dejection, and unhappiness
      b. Dementia is a global, cognitive decline in thinking.
      c. Difference between a depresion which mimics dementia is its' symptomatic presentation.
         - If depression is suspected, treat depression.

G. Multi-Infarct Dementia
   1. Assess for diagnostic specificty; Hachinski criteria can be helpful (Hachinski et al, 1975)
      - A screening instrument to document Transient Ischemic Attacks (TIA's) and ischemic vascular disease.
      - The higher the score, the more suggestive of multi-infarct dementia
   2. Assess for hypertension, spotty cognitive deficits, reliability, depressive symptoms and step wise determination

H. Diagnostic Evaluation
   1. Screening instruments
      a. Mini-Mental Status Examination (MMSE)
      b. ADL and IADL

c. History, physical and mental status exams

d. Laboratory tests; CBC with differential, Chem 18, Thyroid panel incl. TSH, B12, Folate, PSA, RPR, VDRL, Gunderson Lyme test and Drug levels if appropriate

e. Neuroimaging (e.g., MRI, CT scan) Chest X-Ray, EKG

f. Functional examination

g. Mnemonic for evaluation
- D rugs
- E motional disorder
- M etabolic disorder
- E ars, eyes - perception
- N utrition and/or normal pressure hydrocephalus
- T umors/toxins
- I nfection
- A rteriosclerosis/atherosclerosis
- S undowners' syndrome

h. Autopsy

2. Communication Disturbances

a. Expressive aphasia -the individual has difficulty saying what he/she wants to say; grasping for words

b. Receptive aphasia -the individual has difficulty in understanding what is being said to him/her

c. Global aphasia-Receptive and Expressive

I. Treatment
- Currently there are numerus drug studies in progress. Cognex (Tacrine HCL) is a cholines-terase inhibitor and can be helpful in delaying the progression of AD in some cases.

J. Issues in Care

1. Safety and supervision

2. Nutrition/Hydration

3. Activities and stimulation

4. Bowel and bladder programs
5. Fall prevention
6. Decision-making
   - Surrogate management options
   - Financial, ethical, legal issues
   - Aggressiveness of care for end of life or catastrophic illness
7. Family distress
   - Caregiver burnout in the form of fatigue, irritability, stress, depression
   - Referral to medical, mental health resources may be indicated

K. Alternative care
   1. In home with community/family support
      a. Information, Education
      b. Alzheimer's Association
      c. Support groups
   2. Adult day care
   3. Respite
   4. Placement
      - Discuss decision-making process
      - Discuss previously made promises, i.e., "I will never put you in a nursing home."
      - Cultural and religious beliefs
   5. Referral

IX. General Principles of Nursing Intervention

A. Benefits of thorough assessment

1. Development of a high level of differentiation of symptoms that express stress and psychiatric disorders including change in functioning, and activities.

2. Rule out physical illness, acute infection, poly-pharmacy, drug interactions and side effects, social-environmental disruptions

3. Identify the symptoms

4. Define the degree of distress

5. Determine approach depending on acuteness and safety

6. Determine treatment or treatment combination, i.e.

   a. Supportive therapy

   b. Psychotherapy

   c. Behavioral therapy

   d. Cognitive testing

   e. Family interactions

   f. Psychosocial support

   g. Community resources

   h. Placement issues

   i. Need for hospitalization

7. Documentation issues

   a. Psychotic symptoms, organic agitation

   b. Catastrophic reactions

   c. Effectiveness of psychotropic meds

   d. Depressive symptoms; antidepressant agents
      - May take 10-14 days for therapeutic levels to be reached

e. For bipolar disorders, effectiveness of lithium

f. Use of antipsychotics for severe distress, agitation, thought disorders.

g. Use of anxiolytics and consideration to addictive properties. Effectiveness of behavioral approaches, muscle relaxation, guided imagery, and biofeedback for mild to severe anxiety

8. Nurse/Client interactions

a. Allow client to ventialte feelings related to symptoms and situation.

b. Give permission to express/feel anger, fear, loss or share feelings

c. Encouragement and non-judgmental attitude toward expressions of feelings

d. Use of communication techniques, such as clarification, verbal clues (furthering, para-phrasing, open and closed-ended questions) summarizing and interpretation may be indicated

e. Exploration of feelings of dependency and helplessness. Help client find ways verbally and in practice to feel more independent and less helpless by defining tasks that can be accomplished and successfully built upon. The goal should be to establish a hierarchy of successful behavior.

f. Help client to feel mastery and control for one's life by insuring options and choices. The goal is to provide new opportunities to maintain autonomy and make decisions.

Conclusion

There are situations where specific stressors can be eliminated but more often stress has broad reaching ramifications, e.g., widowhood involves not only grieving but loss of a partner, companionship, income, housing, social network, etc.

The elderly are at high risk for successive losses and challenges which affront their coping abilities. The nurse must keep a high index of suspicion for symptoms of emotional distress, psychiatric and cognitive disorders and offer aggressive and comprehensive evaluation and treatment options.

Unit 1 - Chapter 5

The High Risk Profile

I. Frail elderly

A. Fraility

1. Defined by Webster as having a 'delicate condition.'

2. There are increasing numbers of individuals reaching the age of 100 each year.
   - In 1990, this number reached 36,000.

3. 80% of this population is female; 20% are male

4. Diminishing ability to cope with changes in health, environment, and an eroding social support system lead to fraility.

5. Paradoxically, the strength and resilience of this population which has carried them into this group of 'old old,' are the very characteristics which also make them 'frail.'

   -This select group typically has a stronger genetic makeup, healthier lifestyle and an over all adaptive response to the aging process.

6. Physiologically, frail individuals manifest reduced physical capacity, neurologic control, poor mechanical performance and decreased metabolism.

7. Studies show that fraility may be the accumulated effect of acute insults to the individual, such as illness, injury and catastrophic events which lead to change in life-style and immobility.

B. Hardiness vs. Frailty

There have been studies which have looked at the 'hardiness' of individuals as they age. The following are predominant characteristics;

1. Feelings of control

2. Deep committments to something or someone

3. The enjoyment of a challenge

C. Prevention of fraility

   1. Monitoring key physiologic indicators of fraility; i.e. disease, advanced age, known risk factors

   2. Prevention of acute and subacute physiologic loss

   3. Prediction of episodes of physiologic loss and the reduction of maladaptation to changes in health

   4. Removal of obstacles to recovery once physiolgic loss has occurred.

II. Risk factors

A. Iatrogenesis

   - A term usually used to describe the deteriorating health of an elderly individual
   Common factors which lead to iatrogenesis;

   1. Hospitalization

   2. Polypharmacy

   3. Ill effects of aging which lead to deterioation and functional decline

B. Areas of dysfunction which lead to iatrogenesis

   1. Immobility

   2. Instability

   3. Incontinence

   4. Intellectual impairment

   5. Infection

   6. Impairment of vision and hearing

   7. Irritable colon

   8. Isolation (depression)

   9. Inanition (malnutrition)

   10. Impecunity (poverty)

11. Insomnia

12. Immune deficiency

13. Impotence

C. Implications of Iatrogenesis
- "The least desirable outcome of medical care is to decrease the patient's health as a result of contact with the care system."
1. Inaccurate labeling or over diagnosing occurs when generalizations are made about a singular problem, creating an impression of overall physiologic or functional ability.
   - An isolated incidence of incontinence or confusion may dictate a plan of care which may assume chronic problems and inability to maintain self.
2. Careful evaluation is a critical element in care-planning, to avoid inappropriate measures which could adversely affect short and long term goals.
3. It is the nurse who provides the psychosocial input in addition to the physical findings to determine that which is in the client's best interests.

D. Theories of iatrogenesis
1. Iatrogenesis is less likely with factors such as a healthy mental status, positive adaptation to aging, and an active lifestyle.
2. When loss occurs frequently and without time for recovery, the individual's coping mechanisms and resilience are diminished.
3. Loneliness alone, can lead to deterioration in self-perception and subsequently self-care.
4. Physiologic decline can precipitate loss of one's independence and a sense of well-being
5. Response to illness may be altered if the individual's self-worth has been affected adversely.
6. The elderly undergo perhaps more psychosocial stressors than any other age group, dealing with several major

events concurrently; i.e. psychosocial stressors, fear, loneliness, physical deterioration, and loss of loved ones.

7. These types of events require stamina, perserverance and flexibility, which are difficult at best, even for a healthy individual.

8. The older, frail individual must live with challenges, changes and losses.

III. Nutritional concerns

A. Nutritional needs

1. Longitudinal studies have examined dietary variables which are predictive of chronic disease, disability and mortality.

    - Frail elderly living independently are at highest risk of hunger and malnutrition
    - In addition, underrecognition and treatment of poor nutritional habits leads to increased morbidity.

2. Weight loss and protein-calorie malnutrition are common problems.

3. Malnutrition occurs in both under weight and over weight individuals.

4. Poor nutritional content of meals and snacks as well as inadequate calories leads to dietary insufficiency.[4]

B. Characteristics of the malnourished elderly individual living at home

1. Eccentricity

2. Isolation/homebound

3. Poor self-esteem and self-care routines

4. Living in poverty

    - Home-delivered meals have been beneficial for many, but the problems still exist for the geographically isolated.

C. Characteristics of the malnourished elderly individual in the nursing home
   1. Those with severe physical disorders
      - This includes those with swallowing difficulties, digestive disorders and neurologic damage
   2. Those with severe mental disorders
      - This includes those with dementia, depression, and decreased consciousness
   3. Studies have determined that clients with late stage Alzheimer's Disease, often suffer additionally from cachexia, despite high caloric intake.

D. Malnutrition in the elderly
   1. Defined as having deficiencies of:
      - Potassium, Magnesium, Vit. D. and Vit. B_6,
   2. Less than 13g/dl Hgb for males and 12g/dl for females.
   3. Serum albumin levels of less than 3.5 mg/dl, suggests depletion of visceral protein
   4. Cholesterol levels of less than 156 mg/dl are predictive of mortality
   5. Malnutrition is more than twice as common in subjects of 80 years or more, than in younger patients
   6. Signs of malnutrition:
      a. Scurvy
      b. Osteomalacia
      c. Nutritional anemia
   7. Medical factors related to malnutrition:
      a. History of partial gastrectomy
      b. Chronic bronchitis
      c. Emphysema
      d. Depression
      e. Difficulty swallowing

f. Poor fitting or absent dentures
   g. Poor caloric intake in response to wound healing after surgery, burns, or with multiple pressure ulcers
E. Causes of anemia:
   1. Chronic renal failure
   2. Metastatic carcinomas
   3. Gastrointestinal bleeding
   4. Infection
F. Theories of obesity in the eldelry:
   1. Failure to reduce food intake in response to diminished energy expenditure
   2. Overeating due to boredom, lack of a daily routine,
   3. Large meals and snacks
   4. Lack of knowledge of healthy dietary habits
   5. Drugs which increase appetite such as tranquilizers, lithium and steroids

   (See figure 1.)
G. Consequences of obesity
   1. Obesity has a direct effect on morbidity and mortality in the elderly client.
   2. In addition to the added insult to the aged cardiovascular system, respiratory effort may be compromised due to increased fatty tissue and breast size.
   3. Inspiratory and expiratory efforts are both impaired.
   4. There is evidence of immobility due to exaggerated arthritic joints with resultant skin breakdown.
   5. Excessive weight limits the individual's activity level, reducing calorie expenditure and increasing fatiguability.
   6. Orthopedic physicians see thousands of elderly individuals annually with knee, back and joint related pain, as a result of excess weight.

Demographic and Medical Variables Related to Obesity in Elderly Persons	
Variable	**Risk Factor**
Age	Les than 75 years
Sex	Females > males
Socioeconomic status (SES)	Low SES > high SES in females
	High SES > low SES in males
Education	Less than 12th grade
History	Past obesity
	Past repeated attempts to diet
	Lack of physical exercise
Diseases	Maturity-onset diabetes
	Hypertension
	Osteoarthritis (with symptoms related to weight-bearing joints
	Abdominal hernia
	Varicose veins · stasis dermatitis and ulcers
	Gall bladder disease
	Gout
	Psychiatric, neurological, musculoskeletal and other diseases causing confinement to wheelchair or bed*

Drugs: Hyperphagic agents, including phenothiazine and benzodiazepine tranquilizers and lithium carbonate as well as sedatives such as barbiturates.

Drugs used in the treatment of obesity: including amphetamines, thyroid hormones.

Drugs used in the treatment of diseases complicating obesity: including oral hypoglycemic agents, diuretics, other antihypertensive drugs, and non-narcotic analgesics used to treat diabetes, hypertension, osteoarthritis, and gout, respectively.

---

*Obese wheelchair or bedfast elderly patients are those who maintain food energy intake in exces of their needs and do not have diseases which cause energy wastage.

Figure 1

  H. Solutions to obesity

    1. Nutritionists agree that a diet with as few as 600 calories and reduced fat content is one of the most effective solutions to obesity in the older adult.

    2. The use of anorectic drugs, including amphetamines is inappropriate in the elderly, producing adverse effects such as insomnia, excitement, elevated blood pressure and tachycardias.

IV. Risk factors in the community

   A. Home and social emergencies

      1. The modern emergency department is often the entry point for elderly patients with social problems, as well as for those with urgent medical needs. (McDonald)

      2. Entry into the hospital is frequently through admission from the emergency department., from acute illness, injury or trauma or exacerbation of chronic disease.

   B. Elders as victims of crime

      1. Elders are frequently victims of crime, due to increased vulnerability and inability to defend against attack or escape from the perpetrator.

      2. Violent crimes against the elderly are on the increase.

      3. Neighborhood thieves, door-to-door salespeople, and scheming financial investors find the elderly to be 'easy targets.'

      4. The elderly have stronger cultural beliefs regarding trust of strangers.

      5. The older victim typically has difficulty differentiating between a valid transaction and a 'scam.'

      6. Perpetrators of crime perceive the older adult to carry excessive amounts of cash and have more valuables within the home.

      7. Increasingly, a victim of family abuse; physical, psychological and financial.

      8. Falls and other types of trauma are frequent in the home setting.

   C. Risk for injury

      1. Visual, auditory, tactile impairment

      2. Osteoporotic changes

      3. Urinary frequency

      4. Impaired balance

5. Orthostatic changes
6. Decreased mobility, agility
7. Syncope due to cardiovascular changes
8. Increasing age
9. Fear of falling
10. Gait disorders
11. Improper fitting foot wear
12. Loose floor coverings i.e. throw rugs

D. Complications of injury
   1. Rhabdomyolysis
      - Defined as injury which occurs after prolonged periods of immobilization, resulting in ischemic tissue at the site of injury.
      - Damage to tissue occurs from necrosis to striated muscle.
      - In addition, fragility of tissue and impaired circulation increase risk for severe consequences.
      - The elderly are at risk after falls, due to altered consciousness, inability to get immediate assistance and prolonged healing potential.
      - Pressure ulcer development is common.
   2. Treatment after tissue injury
      - Fluid replacement to assure clearance of myoglobin from the urine;
      - Mannitol to improve renal perfusion;
      - Treating hyperkalemia;
      - Treating local injury.

Predisposing Risk Factors and Potential Interventions

Risk Factor	Potential Interventions
Sensory	
Vision: close-range and distance perception, dark adaptation	Appropriate refraction; surgery; medications; goo dlighting
Hearing	Cerumen removal; hearing aid
Vestibular	
Drugs, previous infections, surgery, benign positional vertigo	Avoidance of toxic drugs; surgery, balance exercises, good lighting
Proprioceptive	
Peripheral nerves, spinal cord	Treatment of underlying disease; good lighting; appropriate walking aid and footwear
Cervical: arthritis, spondylosis	Balance exercises; surgery
Central neurologic	
Any central nervous system disease impairing problem solving and judgment	Treatment of underlying disease; supervised, structured, safe environment
Musculoskeletal	
Arthritides, especially lower extremities	Medical and possibly surgical treatment of underlying disease
Muscle weakness, contractures	Strengthening exercixes; balance and gait training, appropriate adaptive devices
Foot disorders; bunions, callouses, deformities	Podiatry; appropriate footwear
Systemic diseases	
Postural hypotension	Hydration; lowest effective dosage of necessary medications; reconditioning exercises; elevation of head of bed; stockings
Cardiac, respiratory metabolic disesases	Treatment of underlying diseases
Depression	Careful consideration to risk/benefit ratio of antidepressant medication
Medications	
All -- especially sedating medications	Lowest effective dosage of essential medications, starting low and increasing slowly

Figure 2

Hazzard, W.; Biermon, E. Bloss, J., Principles of Geriatric Medicine and Gerontology, McGrqw Hlll, 1994

E. Other injuries noted to occur frequently among the elderly
   1. Burns
   2. Suffocation
   3. Poisoning
   4. Scalding
   5. Electric shock
   6. Drowning
   7. Thermal injury, heat stroke, or hypothermia
   8. Driving accidents
F. Driving
   1. Age-related changes including sensory, visual impairment, diminished reaction time, decreased physical agility, and altered hearing, make driving a hazardous activity.
   2. Studies indicate a decline in driving ability at age 75 with a dramatic decrease in ability after age 85.
   3. Factors related to the elder drivers' resistance to stop driving:
      - Need for independence
      - Failure of family to evaluate driving skills
      - Failure to relinquish car keys
   4. Tests reveal that individuals over the age of 85 frequently experience:
      a. Impaired recognition of unexpected vehicles
      b. Inability to maintain speed limit, especially on fast-moving highways
      c. Difficulty reading road signs and other changes in the road i.e. detours, barriers, narrowing.
   5. Those with a dementing illness such as Alzheimer's Disease have documented difficulty with perception and judgement while driving.

6. Recommendations for the elder driver

   a. Avoid night driving

   b. Avoid driving under hazardous conditions i.e. snow, fog, storms

   c. Use sensory aids, such as glasses, hearing aids

   d. Be aware of medication effects or alcohol consumption

   e. Plan frequent rest and stretch periods for long trips

   f. Assure proper maintenance of vehicle

   g. Carry emergency numbers for accessibility should the driver become ill or injured

V. **Alcoholism in the elderly**

   A. Characteristics of the eldelry drinker

      1. Approximately 10% of those over the age of 65 have a drinking problem

      2. Alcoholism is usually under-recognized due to social isolation

      3. The older drinker is usually widowed, divorced or separated

      4. More likely to be male

      5. There may be a history of organic brain disease and a complicated medical history

      6. This is the third most common cause of mental impairment, in addition to dementia and neurosis

   B. Psychosocial contributing factors

      1. Poor adjustment to retirement

      2. Significant losses; spouse, home, financial, close friends

      3. Insomnia

      4. Pain

      5. Depression

6. Anxiety and loneliness
7. May be a factor in suicidal attempts
C. Elders at greater risk for alcoholism
   1. Increased sensitivity to alcohol
   2. Decreased lean body mass
   3. Decreased total body water
   4. Impaired liver and kidney function
D. Difficulty with diagnosis due to
   1. Confusion
   2. Disorientation
   3. Blackouts
   4. History of falls
   5. Cardiomyopathy with poor oxygenation
   6. Hypertension
   7. Poor physical tolerance
   8. Vitamin deficiency
   9. Gastritis
   10. Cirrhosis
   11. Hypoglycemia
   12. Hyperlipidemia
   13. Hyperuricemia
   14. Decreased sexual function
   15. Increased bone loss
   16. Anemia
   17. Folate deficiency
   18. Drug adverse reactions

19. Loss of weight or malnutrition

20. Skin ulcers

21. Self-neglect

22. Depression

E. Issues to consider with the elderly alcoholic

1. Explore social issues which may be contributing; loneliness, financial concerns, etc.

2. Recommend a complete physical exam to rule out any masked disease

3. Seek resources for referral

4. Be aware of withdrawl symptoms and be prepared to treat with short-acting benzodiazepines

5. Avoid cold and cough medicaitons which have alcohol content

VI. Medical/institutional risks

A. Delayed recognition of infection in the home or within an institution is one of the greatest clinical risks for the eldelry patient. Commonly under-diagnosed conditions

1. Cholecystitis

2. Appendicitis

3. Intra-abdominal sepsis secondary to diverticulitis or bowel cancer

4. Meningitis

5. Endocarditis

6. Tuberculosis

B. In addition, delayed recognition of smaller scale infections, such as UTI, (urinary tract infection) can also become problematic when missed during the initial exam.

C. Diseases with higher fatality rates
- Influenza
- Pneumococcal, pneumonia and bacteremia
- Bacterial meningitis
- Gram-negative pneumonia

D. Institutionalization can be a watershed event for many, opening the door to many adverse occurrences.

E. Loss of independence and autonomy as well as physical and psychological decline are inevitable when acute illness results in hospitalization.

F. Problematic behaviors seen when loss of control over body and environment occur
  1. Loss of physical strength due to inactivity
  2. Risk for skin ulcers, decubiti
  3. Nosocomial infection
  4. Social isolation
  5. Sleep pattern disturbances
  6. Risk for abuse or neglect by care providers
  7. Financial burden or impoverishment

VII. HIV/AIDs in the elderly

A. An unlikely population at risk
  1. There is growing concern about this misdiagnosed disease in the elderly
  2. Sexual transmission and transfusion are the most frequent methods of acquisition
  3. Recipients of blood products before 1985
  4. Spouses of those recipients
  5. Persons who participate in unprotected anal or vaginal intercourse outside of a monogamous relationship.

B. Other risk factors for HIV infection in this population
   1. Infrequent use of condoms, due to absence of pregnancy risk
   2. Underestimated sexual activity of elders
   3. Frequent involvement of elderly men with prostitution
   4. Greater numbers of elder men involved in homosexual relationships
   5. Lack of knowledge or failure to recognize risk
C. Presenting complaints which may mask accurate diagnosis
   1. Decreased platelet count
   2. History of diarrhea
   3. Confusion
   4. Weight loss
   5. Apathy
   6. Loss of balance
   7. Leg weakness
   8. Tremors, seizures
   9. Fatigue
   10. Pneumonia
   11. Malnutrition
   12. Dementia with symptoms similar to Alzheimer's Disease
D. Complications include
   1. Decreased resistance to infection
   2. Increased risk for skin breakdown
   3. Frequency and severity of pneumonia
   4. Early immobility with resultant weakness
   5. Increased risk for opportunistic infection

VIII. Dementia/delirium/depression

Studies point to the fact that the longer one lives, the greater is one's chance for developing some form of dementia

A. Dementia is defined as global decline in cognitive function, including memory, language, spatial, or temporal orientation, judgement, and abstract thought.

1. 25% of those between the ages of 65 and 85 are predicted to develop some form of dementia

2. Approximately 50% of those over the age 85 will have symptoms of a dementing disease

3. Recognizable signs of dementia

   a. Global changes in cognition

   b. Insidious memory changes

   c. Speech pattern changes

   d. Visuospatial changes

   e. Apraxia

   f. Alterations in social graces

   g. Paranoia-delusions

   h. Sleep pattern changes

   i. Diminished ability to manage self-care

4. Dementia-type symptoms occur with,

   a. Parkinson's Disease

   b. Huntington's Chorea

   c. Intoxication/ Alcoholism

   d. Infection

   e. Metabolic/Nutritional disorders including dehydration or poor intake of adequate fluids

   f. Neurogenic lesions

g. Depression (pseudementia)
   h. Acute onset of illness
5. Many causes of dementia are reversible, although accurate diagnosis is critical
6. Treatable causes of dementia;
   a. Drugs
   b. Post-anesthesia symptoms
   c. Hypothyroidism
   d. Hyperthyroidism
   e. Hypoglycemia
   f. Vit B_{12} or folate deficiency
   g. Subdural hematoma
   h. Liver failure
   i. Normal pressure hydrocephalus
   j. Stroke
   k. CNS infection
   l. Generalized infections
   m. Cerebral neoplasms
   n. Renal failure
   o. Ethanol abuse
   p. Hypoxia
   q. Hypercalcemia
   r. Vasculitis
   s. Cardiopulmonary disorders
   t. Anemia
   u. Korsakoff's psychosis

7. Irreversible causes of dementia;

   a. Alzheimer's Disease

   b. Pick's Disease

   c. Jacob-Cruetzfeld's Disease

   d. Parkinson's Disease

   e. Huntington's Chorea

B. Delirium

   Delirium is defined as an acute organic brain syndrome manifested by an attentional deficit, rambling or incoherent speech. It is also known as an acute confusional state.

   1. Delirium is often overlooked or unrecognized by many physicians although approximately 50% of patients over the age of 70 on a given medical-surgical unit show some signs of delirium.

   2. Accurate diagnosis of delirium must include at least two of the following:

      a. Reduced level of conscioiusness

      b. Perceptual disturbances; misinterpretations, illusions, hallucinations

      c. Disturbance of sleep-wake cycle with insomnia

      d. Change in psychomotor activity

      e. Disorientation to time, place or person

      f. Memory impairment.

   3. Factors which precipitate delirium

      a. Metabolic disease

      b. Infection

      c. Endocrine disorders

      d. Cardio-respiratory distress

      e. Mass lesions

f. Trauma
  g. Stroke
  h. Toxic substances
  i. Withdrawl from drugs
  j. Depression
  k. Post-anesthesia reaction
  l. Sensory deficits
  m. Psychosocial distress
  n. Alcohol withdrawl
 4. Immediate treatment for delirium includes:
  a. Treatment of underlying acute illness
  b. Appropriate nutrition and hydration
  c. Discontinuance of unnecessary drugs
  d. Comfort measures in the form of reassurance, quiet environment, minimal stimulation
C. Depression
 1. Depression is defined as feelings of sadness, dejection, and unhappiness which result in long periods of apathy, anxiety, loss of appetite, sleep disturbance and thoughts of death or suicide;
 2. This disease process leads to disrupted thought processes, impaired communicatio and sensory dysfuntion;
 3. The most common reason elderly persons seek psychiatric help;
 4. Depression may be chronic or intermittent;
 5. It may accompany life transitions creating an adjustment disorder;

6. Depression often precludes suicidal ideations with feelings of hopelessness, helplessness and despondency.

IX. Death

The image of a dying patient usually brings to mind that of the frail old person, oblivious to the fast-paced high technical world of modern medicine. Dying patients often feel despair and loneliness, even in bustling institutions of health. The research of Dr. E. Kübler-Ross led health care professionals to a better understanding of the needs of the dying patient and his family. Attitudes related to the dying process experienced by the older adult are in opposition to those previously described by Dr. Ross. Anger, denial and hopelessnesss are not necessarily felt as these clients face their final hour.

A. Physical changes that occur during the dying process

1. Cardiovascular changes include decreased peripheral circulation resulting in skin color changes, mottling, coolness and cyanosis.

2. Respiratory alterations mean decreased ability for the lungs to adequately ventilate, resulting in an increased accumulation of fluid in the bronchioles. Decreased ability to clear congestion as well as an irregular respiratory pattern can lead to periods of anoxia. Dyspnea occurs in conjunction with cardiovascular decline, resulting in prolonged periods of apnea and Cheyne-Stokes breathing patterns. Hypoxemia occurs as a result of poor oxygenation.

3. The gastrointestinal tract looses motility, with decreased appetite, anorexia, intestinal blockage and bloating. Dysphagia occurs as the involuntary swallowing musculature looses tone.

4. Diminished blood flow to the kidneys means decreased elevated blood urea nitrogen levels, and urosepsis. Sphincter control is lost, urine becomes amber in color and foul-smelling.

5. Neurologic changes occur due to poor oxygenation, decreased cerebral blood flow and synaptic alterations. Disorientation, lethargy and delirium occur as levels of consciousness decrease.

	Men	Women	Men	Women
	75-84		85 and older	
Heart disease	3239	2122	7830	6810
Malignancies	1861	982	2528	1292
Cerebrovascular Accident (CVA)	603	523	1625	1738
Chronic opstructive pulmonary disease (COPD)	504	197	777	245
Pneumonia and flu	352	199	1428	1006
Accidents	143	84	375	225
Diabetes	127	123	229	219
Suicide	57	7	60	5
Liver disease	44	25	34	14

Nine Most Common Causes of Death Among Persons 75 Years to 84 Years and Older by Frequency of Occurrence per 100,000 Population of that Age Group

From U.S. Bureau of the Census: 1991. *Statistical abstract of the United States*, 111th ed., U.S. Government Printing Office, Washington, D.C.

Figure 3

    B. The needs of the dying patient

        1. Freedom from pain

        2. Freedom from loneliness

        3. Conservation of energy

        4. Maintenance of self-esteem

        5. Reconciliation.

    C. Comfort measures for the dying patient

        1. Provide companionship, especially if families or friends are not available

        2. Provide pain relief as directed by physician orders and as tolerated

3. Provide hydration as tolerated to avoid drying of mucous membranes, including artificial tears

4. Keep environment quiet, softly lit, minimal stimulation

5. Provide repositioning, frequent skin care and protection from pressure areas and breakdown.

6. Offer lip balms, moisturizing lotions, soothing creams as needed

7. Daily bed baths to remove body odor, perspiration and soiling from incontinence

8. Provide comforting conversation, touch, i.e. "I'm here if you need something," "I care about you," "You're a very special person."

9. Offer pastoral support if desired. (Even families who have not previously expressed religious preferences, often choose pastoral support during the end stages of life.)

10. Allow family and friends to remain nearby 24 hours per day. This allows those to begin the grieving process and to express final words to the dying patient.

References

Ebersole & Hess. *Toward Healthy Aging*. Mosby, Inc. (1994)

Kane, Robert., Ouslander, Abrass. *Essentials of Clinical Geriatrics* McGraw Hill (1989)

Schuerman, Debra. "Clinical Concerns: Aids in the Elderly" *Journal of Gerontologic Nursing*, Vol 20 #7 (7/94)

Johnson, Jerry. "Delirium in the Elderly" *Emergency Clinics of North America*, Vol 8 #2; W.B. Saunders, Pub.

Roe, Daphne. *Geriatric Nutrition* (1994)

Roe, Daphne. "Demographics and Medical Variables Regarding Obesity" *Geriatric Nutrition*. Prentice Hall

Hazzard, W., Bierman, E., Bloss, J. "Principle of Geriatric Medicine and Gerontology" *Predisposing Risk Factors and Potential Interventions*; McGraw Hill, (1994)

"Nine Most Common Causes of Death". U.S. Bureau of the Census

Morley, John. "Conditions Associated with Poor Nutrient Intake" " SCALES Protocol for Evaluating Risk of Malnutrition" *Resident and Staff Physician*, Vol 39, #3

Unit 2

The Elderly American; Less Than Optimal Health

Unit 2 - Chapter 1

Ethical Dilemmas

Advanced technology and its application in our health care institutions poses one of the most complicated series of ethical dilemmas of the '90's. Our efforts to maintain life at both ends of the spectrum at all costs places a burden on families, government, and care providers. Recent legislation regarding 'end of life' choices has had a monumental impace on not only the extent of health care one wishes to receive, but also the issue of surrogate decision-making. In addition nationally publicized dramas of famlies torn with difficult decisions regarding loved ones who have suffered irreversible brain damage from traumatic injury has heightened public awareness of the critical nature of discussing personal philosophies about extending life beyond reasonable expectations.

I. Irreversible brain damage

A. There is now a growing population of individuals with a condition known as persistent vegetative state, or persistent unconsciousness.

1. This condition is caused from damage to the brain or advanced disease which results in an irreversible condition with no expectation of recovery.

2. There is global cognitive dysfunction without evidence of purposeful actvitity, meaningful communication, pain or pleasure.

3. Sensory response is absent.

4. There is no attempt to perform activities of daily living, including feeding, toileting, even turning oneself in bed.

5. Cardiac and respiratory function may be normal, thereby keeping the individual's physical health reasonably stable, as long as artificial nutrition and hydration are supplied.

6. There are more than 10,000 people in this country in a persistent vegetative state, at a cost of more than $50,000/patient/year.

7. The emotional and financial burden to the famlies is devastating, leaving psychological scars for a lifetime.

Without 'clear and convincing' evidence of personal wishes for this type of catastrophic event, it is difficult for anyone to reach a decision regarding witholding or withdrawing extraordinary measures for people in persistent unconsciousness.

II. Advanced decision making

A. Discussion of life-threatening scenarios

1. Considered by most to be difficult and morbid

2. Not making a decision regarding personal wishes is in itself a decision to accept the full extent of medical technology

3. The burden of decision-making often falls to the survivors of the individual

   - Often these family members are not fully informed nor have they discussed these types of scenarios with the victim

4. Choices of this nature are best made in non-threatening situations, yet in moments of crisis, this becomes an impossibility.

5. For the older individual who may be physical and mental impairment, the decisions are difficult at best, and are then directed to the next of kin.

6. Crisis decision-making if often based on emotions, rather than that which is reasonable and practical.

B. The right of self-determination

1. One of the most important rights possessed by any individual

2. Enacted in 1991 giving individuals the right to make choices regarding 'end of life' decisions.

   - Includes the right to accept or refuse treatment

The Patient Self-Determination Act

Institutions and patients affected by the law (as a condition of Medicare or Medicaid reimbursement, or both)
  Hospitals: all inpatients, at the time of admission
  Skilled nursing facilities: all residents, at the time of admission
  Home Health agencies: all clients, before coming under the care of the agency
  Hospice programs: all patients, at the time hospice care is begun
  Health maintenance organizations: all members, at the time of enrollment

Obligations of health care providers
  Develop and maintain written policies and procedures regarding advance directives
  Provide written information to patients regarding the patient' right (under state law) to accept or refuse medical or surgical treatment and the right to formulate advance directives and regarding the policies of the provider or organization respecting the implementation of such rights
  Document in the medical record whether or not an individual has executed an advance directive
  Ensure compliance with state law regarding patients' advance directives
  Educate staff and the community about advance directives

Obligations of state and federal governments
  Each state, with the assistance of the Department of Health and Human Services, must develop written materials describing the state's laws concerning advance directives
  The Department of Health and Human Services must develop or approve informational materials on advance directives for nationwide distribution to health care providers; develop and implement a national educational campaign concerning advance directives; and mail information to all Social Security recipients concerning advance directives.

Implementation
  Specific regulations for implementing the Act will be developed by the Department of Health and Human Services.
  The provision of the Act will take effect on 1 December 1991

*Adapted from the Omnibus Budget Reconciliation Act (1)

Figure 1

3. The difficulty is not in choosing death over the present state, but rather the dying process.

4. Individuals and those appointed to be proxy-decision makers have the option to choose the full extent of medical technology, or a customized modified version, eliminating that which appears to be futile, or extraordinary.

5. The goal of self-determination is to provide comfort and dignity to the dying individual, regardless of age, financial means, or religious beliefs.

C. Elderly choices

1. It is generally noted that when faced with 'end of life' choices, the elderly clients choices are those of comfort and dignity rather than for aggressive treatments and procedures.

2. This classic situation present an ethical dilemma for nurses and physicians; feelings of compassion yet frustration.

3. Witholding or withdrawing life-sustaining measures brings about comple moral, ethical and legal issues.

4. Discussion of these moral dilemmas is rare between physician and client and therefore falls to the next of kin who must decide between what is realistic and ethically warranted.

   - "Patients are at the mercy of strangers whose roles they do not and may never understand unfamiliar machines and alien routines that seem totally out of step with their own habits."

D. Hospitalization and acute illness

1. Acute care hospitals inevitably must be concerned with the care and management of elderly patients.

2. Though most patients entering the hospital are provided with information regarding Advance Directives and Patient Bill of Rights, time for discussion is rare.

3. Elderly persons in particular fear that overly zealous application of treatments and procedures may subject them to suffering and indignity and their families to financial ruin.

4. Bioethicists often look at the acuity of the disease process and the benefit versus risk of the treatment when medical-ethical questions arise.
    - In the case of infants and children, the parameters are broad with almost no cost or procedure too extravagant to safe the life in question.
5. The scope narrows at the far end of life's spectrum when the chance of a positive outcome without extensive measures and expense is proportionately diminished.
6. Another ethical point of concern surrounds the issue of 'fatal pathology.'
    - This is defined as a condtion which, if left untreated, would eventually lead to a premature death, i.e.cancer of the liver, acute heart disease, etc. despite extensive interventions.
    - In contrast, an individual who has suffered a cerebrovascular accident, (CVA) with loss of speech, memory and inability to perform ADL's is not at risk of immediate death, because the disease is not imminent.

E. Questions to raise when considering 'end of life' decisions
  1. Is there full understanding of the 'Do Not Resuscitate' (DNR) order and its implicatons?
  2. What are the rights of the individual in regards to these issues?
  3. What are the rights and responsibilites of the family?
  4. Is the individual his own 'responsible party' or has someone else been appointed?
  5. What are the personal beliefs and values which may support or prohibit a decision being made?
  6. Is the individual fully informed of the choices?
  7. Has quality of life been taken into consideration?
  8. What are the responsibilities of the health care team to the dying elderly patient?
  9. Are the measures being instituted humane and dignified?

10. Has the individual experssed personal wishes about end of life concerns?

11. Are there other resources i.e. pastoral, social services, etc. which may be called upon to assist in the decision making process?

These questions present a quagmire of ethical dilemmas for those professionals whose basic philosophy dictates curative and restorative measures. These questions have taken on a new urgency due to the increased capacity to sustain life beyond reasonable hope for recovery. At the same time, there is an obligation for health professionals to offer choices to their clients and to adress a systematic approach for decision-making in life and death decisions.

III. Treatment decisions for the elderly

A. Accepted ethical standards for health care professionals

1. One of the basic tenets of the medical profession is "Do No Harm."

2. With this valid belief, life and death are not in direct opposition for the elderly.

3. The obligation exists to provide quality care at both ends of the spectrum; allowing the client the right to life and the right to death.

4. There is a morally relevant difference regarding advanced age, chronic illness and debilitation that requires treatment of the elderly to be less technological and more individualized.

5. Care is based on the physical, psychological and emotional needs as well as the functional abilities or lack thereof.

B. The client's understanding

1. Elderly clients often lack the factual knowledge for good decision-making related to end-of-life care and must rely upon others for accurate and relevant information.

2. The physician entrusted with the authority and having the expertise to guide ethical decision-making is often desen-

sitized to the individual's personal dilemma and must base his advice on information which is also legally encompassing.

3. Failure on the part of the patient to make a decision regarding the extent of care he wishes to receive has profound implications in the subsequent course of events.

C. Treatment decisions for the aged individual should be based on the following:

1. Wishes the individual expressed during his lifetime regarding health care

2. Care that is reasonable, practical and meaningful

3. Wishes expressed by the family which concur with that of the older member

4. Decisions made by the well-informed client and his family cognizant of the facts and issues surrounding prognosis.

5. Financial concerns which may place undue burden on the survivors

6. Precedence of a similar case or cases where age, disease process and prognosis were similar (This if often referred to as substituted judgement; making decisions based on what someone in a similar situation would want or do; i.e. a panel of 85 year olds deciding for another 85 year old what they themselves would want under the same circumstances.)

IV. Documenting decisions

A. Advance directives

1. Though patients have always had choices regarding treatment options, recent legislation has formalized these decisions in the following forms;
   - Advance Directive
   - Durable Power of Attorney for Health Care
   - Power of Attorney in Fact

2. These documents are legally regarded as clear and convincing evidence of the individual's wishes should incompetence limit decision-making ability.

3. Composed while the individual is coherent and competent, these documents provide personalized directions to the family and physician.
4. The proxy appointed in the Directive should understand the personal values of the individual toward life and death.
    - The actual responsbilities of the proxy vary from state to state.

B. Criteria for advance directives
   1. Advance directives, though legally binding, do not need to be drawn up by an attorney, though must be notarized and witnessed to be considered valid.
   2. There are restricitons on employees of health care facilities being designated as 'decision makers' or appointed as Power of Attorney, to prevent an individual (health care employee) from benefitting financially from the health care decision.
   3. These documents are appropriate when the medical condition is not terminal, i.e., death will not occur within a short period of time, and the individual wishes to express specific measures to be either witheld or withdrawn.
   4. Directives may be revoked or changed by the individual at any time
   5. Families and physicians are not legally bound to honor these documents (To date, there has never been a successful lawsuit brought against a physician or individual for providing too much care.)
   6. It is important that these documents become a permanent part of the medical record, with copies being distributed to the family, physician and attorney.
   7. These documents should be updated annually or whenever circumstances warrant a change.

C. Living wills
   1. These are documents which stipualte the wishes of an individual regarding the use of extraordinary measures to prolong life when the medical condition is terminal and the patient can no longer express his own choices.

2. Usually include the words "No CPR" in the case of a catastrophic event.

3. Living wills have limited benefit in that they are in effect only when the patient's condition is terminal, i.e. will die within a short period of time.
   - The specifications are narrow in that they do not allow for the complexities of a disease.

4. In many states, two physicians must certify that the individual is indeed suffering from a terminal illness.

5. It is possible to revoke a living will at any time.

6. As with advance directives, the family and physician are not bound to honor it.

7. Though legally binding, it does not have to be drawn up by an attorney, though should be witnessed and notarized for validation.

8. Living wills should become part of the permanent medical record, with copies given to the family, physician and attorney.

References

Spicker, Stuart F., Ingman, Stanley R. and Lawson, Ian R. *Ethical Dimensions of Geriatric Care: Value Conflict for the 21st Century.* D. Reidel Publishing Co., Dordrecht, Holland

Day, Alice. *Remarkable Survivors: Insights into Successful Aging Among Women.* Urban Institute Press, Washington, DC

Unit 2 - Chapter 2

The Hospitalized Elderly

The number of elderly individuals hospitalized annually has increased over the last decade. Estimates project that persons 65 and older may use about 160 million days of care in short-term hospitals in the year 2000. Currently, more than 40% of acute care hospital beds are occupied by the elderly. The length of stay for persons 85 and older is approximately 12 days, as opposed to only 10.6 days for persons 65 to 85 and only 5 days for those less than 65 years of age. This number will continue to decline because of regulatory agencies, despite the need for 24 hr. acute nursing caring.

More than 80% of elders have at least one chronic condition and many have multiple illnesses. People with chronic illness generally experience exacerbation's frequently, such as respiratory distress, unrelenting chest pain and dehydration. These along with lesser symptoms often mean a stay in the hospital for the elderly individual.

I. **Chronic illness**

    A. The most common chronic illnesses among the aged include:
        1. Coronary heart disease
        2. Osteoporosis
        3. Diabetes Mellitus, Type II
        4. Hypertension

    B. Disease progression
        1. Disease prevention is the key element in planning for the senior adult, with the following benefits;
            a. Fewer hospitalizations
            b. Less frequent episodes of acute illness
            c. Diminished areas of difficulties with chronic disease.
        2. Studies indicate the progression of chronic disease has an adverse effect on quality of life.

3. Increased disability is directly proportionate to increased morbidity and mortality.

4. Health promotion and prevention related activities have shown great benefit, improving one's change for successful aging.

5. Delaying the onset and progression of disease can lead to optimal functioning and preparedness for the challenges of the aging process.

C. Chronic disease and hospitalization

1. Approximately 25% of the elderly have difficulty with activities of daily living and home management due to chronic illness.

2. Hospitalization generally results in a weakened condition, causing further functional decline and deterioration.

II. Assessment of the hospitalized elderly individual

A. Understanding baseline health in the geriatric client

1. Routine testing often points to variations in values for the elderly client.

2. A thorough understanding of the aging process and its effects on the individual can prevent unnecessary treatments, tests and hospitalization

3. Costly and painful diagnostic studies which put the individual at risk for further complications are avoidable.

B. Understanding acute disease in the geriatric client

Masked symptoms and unfamiliar presentation of illness may result in misdiagnosis and under-treatment if viewed as normal consequences of aging.

C. Determination of baseline levels of health

1. Assess physical strengths and weaknesses

2. Assess emotional status

3. Inquire about functional ability and recent changes

4. Utilize the multi-disciplinary team including the rehabilitative therapies and social service.

5. Develop a plan of care which includes the physiologic impairment as well as functional limitations.

D. Complications associated with hospitalization

The elderly are extremely susceptible to other complications that arise during their hospital stay. Iatrogenesis is not uncommon, due to changes in the environment, multiple drug therapies and prolonged immobility. Commonly seen:

1. Adverse toxic drug reactions

2. Malnutrition and dehydration

   (Often due to the withholding of food or fluid for testing purposes, procedures.)

3. Nosocomial infections

4. Pressure ulcers

5. Incontinence

6. Acute confusion

7. Depression

8. Weakness due to prolonged immobilization

III. Acute cardiac conditions in the elderly

A. Cardiovascular disorders

1. Isolated systolic hypertension is the most prominent form in elderly.

   (Defined as systolic blood pressure above 160 mm Hg and diastolic consistently below 90 mm Hg).

2. More than 50% of those over the age of 65 have elevated systolic pressure with or without increase in diastolic pressure. (Increase in systolic and diastolic pressures are a result of decreased elasticity of the vessels and vascular calcium despotism.)

3. Physicians agree that a gradual increase in blood pressure with increasing age is normal.

4. Well-defined relationships exist between:
   a. Elevated blood pressure and stroke
   b. Transient ischemic attacks (TIA)
   c. Coronary artery disease (CAD)
   d. Sudden death
   e. Congestive heart failure (CHF)
   f. Aneurysms
   g. Renal failure
5. Symptoms can include:
   a. Vertigo
   b. Syncope
   c. Headache
   d. Nausea
   e. Vomiting
   f. Loss of equilibrium can result in injury, especially, falls

B. Coronary artery disease

Defined as narrowing of one or more of the coronary arteries, with the following consequences:

1. Decreased oxygen to the myocardium
2. Ischemia
3. Angina
4. Myocardial infarction

   Physiologic changes may be a result of:
   Diabetes
   Hypertension
   Smoking
   A sedentary lifestyle

More than 80% of those over the age of 65 have some form of coronary artery disease.

C. Congestive heart failure

Inability of the heart to supply the body and heart muscle with adequate circulatory volume and pressure. Cardiac insufficiency leads to:

1. Poor oxygenation
2. Decreased blood pressure regulation
3. Fluid and electrolyte imbalance

Common causes of CHF:

1. Hypertension
2. Coronary artery disease
3. Increasing age

It is the number one admitting diagnosis of those over the age of 65. The following symptoms are common;

1. Peripheral edema
2. Fatigue
3. Shortness of breath
4. "Wet" lung sounds
5. Angina

D. Dysrhythmias in the elderly

Alteration in heart rate and rhythm

1. A result of age-related changes in the sinoatrial node and conduction system, including the Bundle of His.
    - Includes decreasing cells in the SA (pacemaker) node
2. May result from increased deposits of adipose and fibrous tissue in the myocardium.
3. Bradycardia
    a. Defined as a rate slower than 60 beat per minute and resulting in hemodynamic instability
    b. Often treated by implantation of a fixed rate pacemaker

        c. Inferior MI, hypothermia, myxedema, or increased intracranial pressure can cause bradycardia
- E. Hypokalemia

    Serum postassium of 3.3 mEq/l or less

    1. May be due to use of diuretics without potassium replacement
    2. May occur with episodes of diarrhea
    3. May be asymptomatic, unless level reaches a critically low level, resulting in ventricular fibrillation and death.
- F. Peripheral vascular disease
    1. Affects the lower extremities in which there is an abnormal narrowing or dilatation of the veins or arteries.
    2. Arterial peripheral disease commonly occurs in men between the ages of 50 - 70 and women after menopause.
- G. Atypical presentation of symptoms common in the elderly
    1. Lightheadedness
    2. Disturbances in gait and balance
    3. Loss of appetite and unexplained weight loss
    4. Inability to concentrate
    5. Changes in personality
    6. Changes in grooming habits
    7. Unusual patterns in urination and defecation
    8. Emotional incontinence
    9. Vague discomfort, bouts of anxiety
    10. Excessive fatigue
    11. Withdrawl from usual sources of pleasure

IV. Respiratory disorders

Any form of respiratory distress, such as that experienced with exertion or pulmonary distress, puts the elderly client at risk for further complications due to a reduced ability to compensate for anoxia (decreased oxygen) or hypercapnia (increased CO_2 level.)

- Normal O_2 levels may be as low as 80% as compared to norms of 92 to 98 % in younger patients.

A. Chronic obstructive pulmonary disease (COPD)

1. Progressive respiratory disease syndrome which may be diagnosed as emphysema, chronic bronchitis or bronchoconstriction

2. Affects approximately 10% of the older population and is the fifth leading cause of death

3. Is responsible for 7 out of every 1000 death in the elderly

4. Can lead to malnutrition from an increase in expended energy from breathing and a resultant decrease of the necessary energy to eat or prepare meals

B. Chronic obstructive bronchitis

1. Defined as an increase in the mucoid bronchial secretions

2. Most commonly seen in men, usually with a long smoking history

3. Disease causes copious secretions to form within the bronchioles necessitating frequent expectoration

4. Prevalence increases with advancing age

C. Asthma

1. Defined as acute reversible episodic obstructive airway disease characterized by resistance in the alveoli

2. Adult onset usually occurs after age 65

3. Physiologic airway resistance either reverts spontaneously or with aerosol treatments.

D. Emphysema
   1. Defined as an increase in the size of the air space distal to the terminal bronchioles.[6]
   2. Characterized by chronic shortness of breath, even in the absence of exertion.

E. Pneumonia
   1. A bacterial or viral infection which settles in pulmonary tissues, causing fever, fatigue and respiratory distress
   2. The elderly are at greatest risk for high incidence of morbidity and mortality when diagnosed with pneumonia.
      - Those over the age of 85 are 5 times more vulnerable than younger adults.
      - Pneumonias are responsible for 25% of the mortality in the aged.
   3. Pneumococcal pneumonias are the most common bacterial respiratory infections of this age group.
   4. 25% - 60% of the elderly are found to have some type of respiratory infection upon autopsy.
   5. Presentation of illness may include:
      - Low grade fever
      - Shortness of breath
      - Weak cough
      - Mental status changes
   6. Aspiration pneumonia is commonly seen in the obtunded adult who has swallowing difficulties, heavily sedated or who may be force fed.
      - Displacement of nasogastric tubes can also lead to aspiration pneumonia.
      - May be the beginning of a terminal event, due to an impaired cough mechanism, impaired immune response and multiplicity of illness.

F. Tuberculosis
   1. Defined as a highly contagious infection which occurs in richly oxygenated tissues, especially the lungs.

2. It is a chronic disease which can result in compromised ability to breath and overall endurance.

3. Vaccination in the elderly may not be effective due to an impaired immunologic response, though Mantoux testing is extremely important.

4. Reinfection with tubercle bacilli is a problem among the elderly whose initial infection is so remote and completely healed that the immune memory of the T cells can be lost.

    a. *Mycobacterium tuberculosis* (M.tb), though treated aggressively during WWII with Isoniazid, can activate in a compromised immune system. (One that has encountered chemotherapy, HIV or advanced age)

5. The Centers for Disease Control have suggested that residents and staff of long term care facilities are at risk for outbreaks of TB and recommend regular Mantoux skin testing.

6. Presentation of symptoms include:

    a. Fever

    b. Night sweats

    c. Weight loss

    d. Cough

    e. Hemoptysis

7. Diagnosis is confirmed by chest X-ray and sputum culture.

V. Gastrointestinal disorders

A. Normal changes that occur with advanced age:

1. Decreased intestinal tract secretions

2. Decreased gastric acid and ptyalin (an enzyme secreted which produces starch)

3. Decreased hydrochloric acid in the stomach

4. Decreased levels of pepsin

5. Decreased fat absorption
6. Decreased ability of the body to absorb vitamins
7. Decreased lipase activity in the digestive tract
8. Decreased peristalsis and the relaxation of the lower esophageal sphincter

B. Diverticular disease
   1. Outpouching of the mucous membranous lining of the bowel through a defect in the muscle layer.
   2. Affects more than 50% of the population over the age of 70.
   3. Symptoms may be minimal, but patients may present to the emergency department with severe pain, due to hemorrhage, abcess or diarrhea.
   4. Symptoms of the disease may be avoided by an increased amount of roughage in the diet, including bran, whole grains, and rice.

C. Ulcerative colitis
   1. Also known as Crohn's disease and ischemic colitis
   2. Occurs more frequently with the aging process
   3. Produces episodes of severe abdominal pain, diarrhea and possible rectal bleeding.

D. Bowel obstruction
   1. Also known as blockage of the intestine
   2. May be simple blockage or a strangulation of the intestine
   3. Usually occurs in the ileum, the narrowest segment
   4. Symptoms include nausea, vomiting, dehydration and severe pain
   5. Emergency surgery is frequently necessary
   6. The mortality in the elderly is high, especially if not correctly diagnosed in the first 24 Hs.

7. Cancer accounts for approximately 80% of obstructions in the large intestine

E. Stress ulcers

1. Ulceration of the gastrointestinal mucosa

2. Characterized by increased acid secretion and rapid stomach emptying

3. Bed-ridden patients frequently develop stress ulcers

4. The mortality for a ruptured stress ulcer is approximately 50%.

5. Treatment includes H_2 receptor antagonists such as Zantac or anticholinergics such as Bentyl, which decrease gastric motility and inhibit gastric secretions

F. Appendicitis

1. Occurs infrequently in the elder adult, but is often misdiagnosed due to similarity of symptoms to more common disorders, such as obstruction or constipation.

2. Peritonitis frequently occurs due to poor tissue perfusion and resistance to infection.

G. Gastrointestinal malignancies

1. Cancer of the colon and rectum are common diseases for the elderly.

2. May be overlooked due to similarity of symptoms, such as vague abdominal pain, constipation, rectal bleeding

3. Symptoms include malaise and weight loss, with changes in mood and cognitive function.

VI. Genitourinary disorders

A. Renal failure

1. Defined as a significant decrease in renal function due to an inability of the kidneys to concentrate and excrete urine, maintain fluid and electrolyte balance or filter nitrogenous wastes.

2. With aging, glomerular tufts, which make up the filtering system, become sclerotic with up to a 12% loss in functional ability by age 70.

3. Up to 50% of hospitalizations for acute renal failure are for clients over the age of 70.

4. Decreased drug elimination by the kidney is the most critical issue in renal failure, resulting in ineffective drug therapy as well as toxicity.

B. Urinary tract infection (UTI)

Hospitalized elderly, especially those who are catheterized pre or post operatively, or who may be immobilized for long periods of time are at risk for UTI.

1. Prevalence of UTI increases with age, becoming the second most common infection in the elderly.

2. Responsible factors include:

    a. Changes in acid-base balance

    b. Inability of the defense mechanisms of the bladder to deal with bacteria

    c. Inefficient micturition due to cystoceles in women and prostatism in men

    d. Open-system indwelling catheters which are infected with bacteria

    e. A warm, moist perineal environment which occurs with clients who wear incontinence protection

3. Presentation may be atypical:

    a. Altered mental status

    b. Nausea, vomiting

    c. Abdominal tenderness

    d. Alterations in respiration

4. Generalized symptoms include:

    a. Low-grade fever

b. Dysuria

c. Frequency

VII. Neurologic disorders

A. Cerebrovascular accident (CVA)

1. Commonly known as stroke, results from hemorrhage within the brain, caused by a rupture of a blood vessel.

2. There can be hemorrhage outside the brain in the subarachnoid space, caused by a ruptured aneurysm.

   - The most common cause of of bleeding in the subarachnoid space is due to intake of prescribed anticoagulants.

3. Stroke can be a result of ischemia as a result of an occlusive thrombi or emboli.

4. Hemorrhagic strokes are most often life threatening, often a consequence of hypertension

5. Thrombotic stroke usually causes damage to the brain, i.e.. paralysis, dysarthria, memory and speech impairment.

6. Mortality from CVA in the elderly is approximately 80%, particularly those caused by hemorrhagic stroke.

7. Signs and symptoms include:

   a. Headache of various degrees, radiating from the back of the head and neck

   b. Nausea, vomiting, dizziness

   c. Confusion, agitation, weakness

   d. Massive cerebral bleeds result in coma and often death.

8. Depression is common after any type of stroke.

B. Transient ischemic attacks (TIA)

1. Brief episodes of focal neurologic dysfunction caused by an ischemic episode which resolves spontaneously

2. 25% of all falls in the elderly are said to be due to TIAs.

3. Frequent TIAs can be a warning of more serious complications.

4. Signs and symptoms may include:

   a. Feelings of confusion

   b. Momentary loss of consciousness

   c. Temporary loss of feeling in extremities

   d. Description of a "shade" coming over one eye

   e. Brief episode of staring and unresponsiveness

C. Intracranial hemorrhage

1. The third most frequent cause of stroke is primarily a result of hypertension or trauma to the head.

2. The bleeding occurs within brain tissue causing displacement and compression.

3. Symptoms include headache, dizziness, epistaxis, mental status changes and acutely, coma and death.

4. Functional improvement is inversely proportional to age.

VII. Hematologic/malignant disorders

A. Anemia

1. A frequent diagnosis among the elderly, ranging from chronic iron deficiency, pernicious anemia (B_{12} deficiency) or folic acid deficiency.

2. Symptoms include complaints of increasing weakness, poor appetite and increased difficulty performing ADLs.

3. Atypical symptoms may include apathy, confusion and depression which may mask the underlying disorder.

4. Dehydration and polycythemia from preexisting disease may limit accuracy of screening diagnosis.

5. Increased hematocrit levels may indicate dehydration.

6. Etiology of iron deficiency:

   a. High intake of aspirin (ASA)

   b. Use of nonsteroidal anti-inflammatory drugs (NSAID)

   c. Peptic ulcer disease

   d. Carcinomas of the colon

   e. Use of anticoagulants

B. Malignancies

   1. The longer a person lives, the more likely that cancer will develop.

   2. Malignancies among the elderly are notuncommon, increasing in frequency with age.

   3. Colon and rectal cancer are among the three most frequent types of cancer found in the over 55 age group.

   4. Theories of autoimmune disorders in the elderly:

      a. Lymphoid depletion and hypoplasia, with thymic atrophy and decreased T-cell function

      b. Suppression of lymphocytes due to diminished thymic function

      c. Decreased functioning of the immune system, with subsequent poor resistance to infection

   5. Adult onset diabetes mellitus may also be considered a disease related to the aging process emanating from immunodeficiencies.

VIII. Elderly in the emergency department

"It is the Emergency Department that will witness the effect of diminished funding for social programs, changes in the length of stay of elderly patients being discharged from in patient hospital beds, shortages of home care resources and changes in the family systems which have historically provided for the supportive care of elderly family members in the home."

A. Demographics
 1. The number of elderly individuals being seen in the emergency department. is increasing each year.
 2. More than 45% of those visiting the ED, over the age of 75 are admitted to the hospital.
 3. The length of stay is usually twice as long for the older client, with a greater number of diagnositic tests.
 4. More likely to be admitted to the ICU
 5. Receive more radiologic and laboratory studies
 6. The elderly are twice as likely to use ambulance services than younger clients.
 7. Incur greater charges
 8. Have more comorbid conditions

B. Characteristics of the elderly emergency department patient
   1. Complexity of medical complaints
   2. Usually from a strained social environment
   3. Very often Medicaid recipient
   4. Largely noncaucasian population
   5. Medical problem is usually related to the limitations of self-care issues, i.e. falling, dehydration, poor nutrition, improper compliance with medications.
   6. Limited transportation for Dr.'s office visits
      - Unnecessary use of ambulance service
   7. Repeat visits are due to unmet social problems, i.e. loneliness, poor support system, unable to follow instructions for self-care.

Causes of Injury by Patient Group

Injury Mechanism	Controls (%) (21 to 64 yr) (N=43)	Elderly (%) (65+ yr) (N=72)	P
Fall	12 (28)	51 (71)	<.0001
Motor vehicle crash	7 (16)	6 (8)	NS
Assault	5 (12)	2 (3)	NS
Work related	9 (21)	0 (0)	NS
Other	10 (23)	13 (18)	NS

Figure 3

C. Admitting complaints
   1. May be more acute in the elderly
   2. Multiple physiologic concerns
   3. Presentation of illness often altered
   4. Polypharmacy and functional impairment often present
   5. Falls or injuries
   6. Exacerbation of a chronic illness

7. Increased edema or other symptoms from CHF

(See figure 4)

Reasons for ED Visit by Patient Group

Category*	No. of Controls (%) (Age 21-64 yr)	No. of Elderly (%) (Age 65+ yr)	P
No personal physician	35 (21) (N=167)	37 (10) (N=389)	<.0005
Referred to ED by physician	34 (20) (N=166)	123 (32) (N=388)	<.01
Too sick to wait for office visit	123 (73) (N=169)	306 (78) (N-394)	NS
Taken to ED from injury site	33 (20) (N=265)	59 (15) (N381)	NS
Care believed better in ED	72 (43) (N-166)	163 (43) (N-383)	NS
Office visits not covered	45 (29) (N=156)	103 (27) (N=377)	NS

*Categories were not mutually exclusive.

Figure 4

    D. Psychosocial Events

        1. Studies have suggested that psychosocial impairment such as loneliness, depression, some sort of abuse or neglect may trigger a visit to the only all night refuge in the neighborhood.

        2. A visit to the emergency department often is a cry for attention from family, physician and friends.

        3. Emergency Department visits almost always constitute some type of follow-up, from family, physician or social services, answering the call for attention.

    E. Drug and chemical abuse

        1. Elders with diminished mental health frequently abuse the psychoactive medications prescribed for them.

2. Those of higher socioeconomic level often misuse analgesics and sedatives.

3. The elderly alcoholic is usually suffering from concomitant depression, as well as physical ill health.

F. Elder abuse

1. The economic stress of living beyond one's expected lifetime is a known factor in the elder abuse theories.

    - Increased financial demands as well as decreasing resources lead to domestic hardships to family and the aging adult.

2. The major types of abuse in the elderly:

    a. Physical...Includes not only infliction of pain on the individual by hitting, kicking, beating, or molesting, but also restraining the individual by tying them to chairs, beds, etc., confining them to beds, closets, or locked areas.

    b. Psychological...Includes threats, isolation, name-calling, humiliation, intimidation and insults.

        - It may be a result of dysfunctional communication within the family.

    c. Financial or material...The deliberate misuse of money or property, including pension, social security, insurance reimbursement or other assets.

    d. Neglect...Occurs when the caregiver fails to provide adequate resources, protection, or other necessities to maintain adequate health and safety.

        - Neglect can be passive, such as ignoring physical and medical needs, or active neglect which includes failure to give medication or food, not tending to personal hygiene or failure to provide safe living conditions.

3. The typical elder abuse victim is:

    a. dependent on others,

    b. female,

    c. over the age of 76,

d. physically or mentally impaired,

   e. a victim of family stress or violence,

   f. impoverished,

   g. widowed,

   h. socially isolated,

   i. a financial burden on others,

   4. Profile of abusers in long-term care:

      a. Care is very demanding

      b. Majority of caregivers are non-professional

      c. Employees have low self-esteem

      d. Low wages are earned for difficult work

      e. High patient to staff ratios

G. Trauma in the elderly

   1. Causes of death in the elder trauma population:

      a. Falls

      b. Thermal injuries
         - Are responsible for approximately 10% of accidental deaths for those over the age of 65

      c. Motor vehicle accidents
         - Are responsible for more than 25% of death in those 65 and over
         - The elderly have the second highest rate of collision, (the highest rate is for those under age 25).

   2. Deterioration in function and chronic disease have been found to be causative factors in accidental injury.

   3. Severity of injury more often results in death in the elderly client than in those younger.

   4. 18% of the older client seen in the emergency department. are there for traumatic injury
      - 25% of the under 65 age group present for trauma.

H. Victims of falls in the emergency department
   1. The likelihood of falls increases with age.
   2. More deaths occur from falls among people age 85 and over.
   3. A non-injury fall may produce debilitating fear and decreased mobility.
   4. Causative factors leading to falls:
      a. Tripping over scatter rugs, furniture, stairs and other objects, such as small pets.
      b. Decreasing sensory perception, loss of peripheral vision
      c. Peripheral neuropathy, leading to decreased sensation in the hands and feet
      d. Decreased visual acuity
      e. Diminished proprioception
      f. Syncope
      g. Postural instability
      h. TIAs
      i. Alcohol ingestion
      j. Associated problems with polypharmacy
      k. Exposure to a new environment, such as occurs in a relocation to an apartment, nursing home or hospital
   5. Common injuries associated with falls:
      a. Fractures of hip, pelvis and/or femur
      b. Colles' fracture of the wrist
      c. Head injury
I. Chronic disease
   1. Increases one's incident for injury

2. Exacerbation of disease which results in momentary loss of consciousness can lead to injury:

   a. Seizure disorder

   b. Cardiac dysrhythmias

   c. Cerebrovascular disease

J. Musculoskeletal system

   1. The most frequently occurring injury to the musculoskeletal system is hip fracture.

   2. Recovery is related to age, previous functional ability and current state of health.

   3. The most common complication is due to prolonged periods of immobility.

   4. Older bones and tissues develop stiffness and loss of motion more quickly.

   5. Pneumonia, pressure ulcers and constipation occur frequently following hip fracture surgery.

   6. Early rehabilitation promotes healing, increased levels of energy and a sense of progress and hope for the client.

K. Fluid and electrolyte balance

   1. The fragile metabolism and inability to compensate for even minor changes in levels of enzymes can lead to serious complications.

   2. Hypokalemia...Serum potassium less than 3.3 mEq/L
      - Common among the elderly due to use of laxatives and diuretics

   3. Hyperkalemia...Serum potassium greater than 5.0mEq/L
      - Occurs with age-related renal changes, renal disease medication toxicity

   4. Hyponatremia.....Decrease in serum sodium concentration to less than 135 mEq/L

5. Malnutrition...Imbalance between the nutrient supply to tissues and the requirements for that nutrient, whether from inadequate dietary intake or defective utilization by the body

L. Sensory alterations

1. Sensory changes occur normally with the aging process.

    a. Diminished vision (presbyopia)

    b. Diminished hearing (presbycusis)

    c. Decreased sense of taste and smell

2. Changes in the environment may be misinterpreted due to mild dementia, sensory changes or memory loss.

3. Sundowning...A term used to describe confusional states which occur toward late afternoon or evening. It is suggested that changes in lighting, or shading at the end of the day may be partly responsible.

4. Common causes of confusion in the hospitalized elderly:

    a. Pneumonia or other fever producing infections

    b. UTIs

    c. Diabetes

    d. Hyperthyroidism

    e. Vitamin B_{12} deficiency

    f. Decrease in red blood cells

    g. Fecal impaction

    h. Elevated temperature

    i. Bladder distension

    j. Dehydration

    k. Relocation anxiety

    l. Narcotics, anesthetics

M. Emergency management issues

1. Physiologic changes as well as psychosocial issues require special considerations in the elderly.

2. Intubation may be difficult if cervical osteoarthritis is present.

3. Laryngeal tissues are more fragile, resulting in damage during ventilatory attempts.

4. If intubation takes place, weaning from the ventilator is often difficult due to decreased pulmonary resilience and diminished tidal volume.

5. Introduction of infection is common, increasing the risk for morbidity.

6. Fluid replacement must be monitored closely to avoid overload in a compromised cardiovascular system.

7. Pressure ulcers, skin tears and ineffective wound healing are common.

8. Ethical and moral issues are critical, providing the individual with choices and dignity when life is in the balance.

IX. Care of the elderly surgical patient

The life expectancy for senior adults continues to rise as medical technology and specialized research bring debilitation into a manageable arena. Without this level of medical interventions, not only would lives end prematurely, but many would lose quality of life in the process. The decision to accept extensive medical treatment, can be a difficult one, and often creates a moral and ethical dilemma.

A. The decision for extensive surgical procedures; Questions to ask:

1. Will the natural course of the disease bring a premature end to this person's life?

2. Will the individual's state of health withstand surgery?

3. If surgery is not chosen, how will quality of life be affected?

4. Will the benefit outweigh the risks?

5. Are there financial resources available that will justify the burden of the procedure?

6. Are there alternatives available that will produce similar results without surgery?

B. Risks with surgery

1. The elderly surgical client is at higher risk for morbidity and mortality.

2. Prophylactic antibiotics should be given when appropriate.

3. Care to avoid hypothermia during surgery is imperative.

4. Extremities and bony prominences should be examined frequently for color, temperature and circulation.
   - Use of mechanical warming devices may be helpful

C. Pre-op surgical assessment

1. Accurate documentation of baseline physical and mental health is critical in determining any normal variations and preexisting conditions.

2. Resilience and rehabilitative potential must be addressed in the plan of care.

3. Multidisciplinary team meetings should evaluate the need for resources once the individual is discharged from the hospital.

D. Physiologic risks pre-operatively

1. Respiratory risks

    a. Decreased vital capacity due to rigidity of the rib cage
       - Expansion ability is limited with increased potential for secondary pneumonia

    b. Potential for decreased oxygen saturation and shallow respiratory effort post-operatively

    c. Surgery to the abdomen produces a compromised respiratory effort.
       - Clients complain of increased incisional pain with post-op turning, coughing and deep breathing.

d. Weaning from ventilatory support may be extended, with increased risk for infection and extreme fatigue ability.

2. Cardiovascular risks

   a. Hypertrophy with decreased elasticity of the myocardium produces diminished cardiac output.

   b. Coronary artery disease and atherocsclerosis resultant poor perfusion can lead to emboli production, infarction and congestive heart failure.

   c. Ischemic episodes can produce a ventricular arrhythmia.

   d. Bradycardia may occur post-anesthesia.

3. Renal risks

   a. Excretion of anesthetic metabolites may be difficult if pre-existing renal insufficiency is present.

      - The duration of activity of any drug is determined by the amount of time the drug remains in the body. Adverse effects from anesthesia in the elderly are common.

   b. Diminished renal perfusion and glomerular filtration rate can be a result of decreased cardiac output.

   c. Brief periods of hypovolemia and hypotension may compromise renal function.

   d. Hemodialysis may be instituted temporarily if there has been an insult to the kidneys.

3. Gastrointestinal risks

   a. Reduction of hydrochloric acid and enzymes, with a resultant decrease in the absorption of drugs can produce;
      - Post-operative bloating
      - Constipation
      - Stress ulcers
      - Wound dehiscence

b. The client may require IV fluids, TPN or other parenteral support for longer periods of time post-operatively until peristalsis and absorption return.

4. Musculoskeletal risks

   a. Post-operative immobility has an exaggerated effect on the elderly individual.

   b. Functional ability deteriorates quickly, proportionate to length of time the client is immobile.

   c. Risk for pressure sores on the heels, elbows, sacrum and pelvic bones is great.
      - Decreased fat distribution on bony prominences as well as poor post-op nutrition increase risk.

   d. Specialized pressure-relieving mattresses, early range of motion and protective devices are strongly recommended during the recovery process.

5. Nutritional risks

   a. Secondary malnutrition and dehydration reduce healing and increase complications during the post-op period.

   b. The client may have decreased nutritional intake prior to hospitalization, due to pain, vomiting, depression, or poor dietary habits.

   c. Post-operative consideration to nutritional needs should include diaphoresis, diuresis, catabolic effects of surgery, medication-producing constipation and diarrhea.

   d. Protein-energy malnutrition (PEM) occurs in previously well-nourished individuals when hospitalized and placed in a starvation regimen because of infection, injury or surgery.

      Symptoms of PEM include:
      - Apathy
      - Weakness
      - Edema
      - Delayed wound healing
      - Intolerance of anesthesia

- Susceptibility to adverse drug reactions
- Impaired cellular immune function
   e. Expected abnormal lab values include;
      - Lymphocytopenia
      - Hypoalbuminemia
6. Cognitive Considerations
   a. Acute confusional states are common, especially among the over 85 age group.
   b. Delirium, as a result of anesthesia, relocation syndrome, or infection occurs frequently.
   c. Confusional states can result from:
      - Sensory overload
      - Memory loss
      - Decreased ability to process information
      - Medication
      - Stress
      - Pain
      - Metabolic imbalance
      - Hypoxia
   d. Thorough baseline assessment from the client and a collateral source should rule out normal variations.
7. Psycho social Factors
   a. Hospitalization becomes traumatic to any individual with physical and cognitive impairment.
   b. Pre-existing factors which may lead to sub-optimal outcomes include:
      - Social isolation
      - Loneliness
      - Residence in a nursing home
      - Infirmity
      - Recent loss of a spouse
      - Depression

c. Optimal outcomes are predicted for:
- Those who are relatively independent
- Those who do not live alone
- Those with supportive family members

X. Iatrogenesis in the Hospital

The nature of most disease processes which put the elderly in the hospital also put them at risk for complications.

A. Pressure ulcers

1. Contributing Factors

    a. Immobility

    b. Age-related skin changes

    c. Malnutrition

    d. Cognitive impairment

    e. Vascular insufficiency

    f. Pressure on bony prominences

    g. Shearing (abrasion to the skin, usually from bed sheets, which occur during turning, repositioning or lifting the client

    h. Friction

    i. Moisture

2. Statistically

    a. When pressure ulcers are listed as the primary discharge diagnosis, the hospitalized mortality rate ranges from 23 to 37%.

    b. 71% of pressure ulcers occur in patients over age 70.

    c. 60,000 persons die annually from ulcer-related complications, including sepsis and osteomyelitis.

    d. 90% occur below the waist.

- e. Low pressure over a long period of time causes more damage, than high pressure over a short period of time.
- f. Moisture (incontinence) leads to a 6% increased risk for ulceration.
- g. 20% of nursing home residents will develop pressure sores at some time.

3. Grades of pressure ulcers
   a. Stage I...Non-blanchable erythema of intact skin. Color does not return after 15 seconds
   b. Stage II...Partial thickness skin loss involving dermis and epidermis
   c. Stage III...Full thickness skin loss, involving damage or necrosis of subcutaneous tissue. Ulcer presents as a deep crater
   d. Stage IV...Full thickness skin loss with extensive destruction, tissue necrosis, damage to muscle, bone or supporting structures

4. Keys to prevention of pressure ulcers
   a. A thorough assessment of risk for skin breakdown
   b. Baseline lab work to determine albumin levels and signs of dehydration
   c. Nutritional assessment to determine caloric and nutrient intake
   d. Regular schedule for turning; usually at two hour intervals, but more often as necessary
   e. Special low air loss mattress products which minimize pressure to bony prominences

5. Treatment
   a. Vitamin C, 500 mg p.o. b.i.d.
   b. Antibiotics i.e. gentamycin, clindamycin

c. Debridement of necrotic tissue to decrease bacterial cell count

   d. Occlusive dressings (Optimal for Stage III)

   e. Collagen wound packing

   f. Surgical intervention with skin flap for Stage III and Stage IV

   g. Moist dressings

B. Incontinence

   1. About 40% of residents in nursing homes and 38% of older women in the community complain of problems with incontinence.

   2. Poorly managed incontinence can lead to severe complications:

      a. Infection (UTI)

      b. Depression

      c. Curtailment of social activities

      d. Premature institutionalization

      e. Increased risk for pressure ulcers (moisture and bacteria near bony prominences)

   3. Patients at risk for incontinence:

      a. Cognitive impairment

      b. Neurologic problems, i.e. stroke, head injury

      c. Back or hip injury

      d. Acute confusional state (surgery, anesthesia)

      e. Medications (calcium channel blockers, diuretics)

      f. Psychological disorders (i.e. depression)

      g. Endocrine disorders (i.e. thyroid disease, diabetes)

      h. Stool impaction

4. Urinary frequency and incontinence may be a sign of UTI. Urinalysis, urine culture, electrolytes, BUN, creatinine and thyroid stimulating hormone should be drawn.

5. Bladder training can be instituted by starting the patient on a regular toileting schedule, monitoring I & O, assuring that assistance is available for the dependent client.

C. Sleep disturbances

1. Hospitalization can exaggerate pre-existing sleep in the elderly.

2. According to studies, total sleep time for the elderly does not change, but there are more periods of wakefulness, and more time spent in bed.

3. Change in environment and daily routines, such as hospitalization, can affect sleep patterns, producing a type of psychosis.

4. Symptoms related to sleep psychosis include:

   a. Delirium

   b. Increased confusion

   c. Agitation

   d. Hallucinations

5. Insomnia, as well as increased periods of sleep may be a sign of impending illness or depression.

6. Treatment includes assessment of normal sleep patterns, ruling out exacerbation of physical or cognitive impairment and creation of a routine and environment which encourages restfulness.

D. Medication toxicity

1. Anatomic and physiologic changes have a critical effect on drug metabolism in the elderly.

2. Age-related changes include:

   a. Decreased body mass

    b. Circulating blood volume

    c. Increased fat deposits

  3. Effects of medication on the elderly:

    a. Slower metabolism

    b. Diminished excretory ability of the kidneys

    c. Increased sensitivity to narcotics and other CNS depressants

E. Infections

  1. Infectious diseases ranging from appendicitis to herpes zoster cause significant morbidity among the elderly.

  2. Delayed recognition of potentially life-threatening infection is a critical problem.

  3. Studies show that older adults suffering from acute abdominal infections usually delay seeking help for 24 to 48 hrs. longer than younger clients with the same complaints

  4. Two of the most prevalent infections causing increased morbidity and mortality;
     - pneumonia
     - influenza

  5. Newly developed immunizations for pneumonia and flu have dramatically reduced the risk for mortality.

  6. Nosocomial infections also account for approximately 10% of the mortality rate among the hospitalized and institutionalized elderly.

  7. *Clostridium difficile* (C. diff.), an intestinal infection which causes persistent diarrhea, is a significant cause of morbidity.

  8. Methycillin resistant staphylococcal aureus (MRSA) occurs frequently in the hospitalized elderly due to decreased immune response, presence of existing infection and increased resistant to antibiotics.

XI. Nursing interventions for the hospitalized elderly

A. Develop an interdisciplinary team approach

1. Perform complete physical, functional and cognitive assessments documenting baseline behaviors.

2. Coordinate timely meetings which support and focus on functional abilities.

3. Encourage patient and family involvement in care issues.

B. Care planning

1. Individualize care-planning to meet specific geronotologic issues.

2. Develop patient teaching plans which support lifestyle changes.

3. Address long term care issues for debilitating illness or injury.

4. Focus on a plan which assists the elderly client to adapt to present health status and impending changes.

XII. Discharge planning

A. Trends

1. Elderly patients are being discharged quicker and sicker.

2. Post-discharge outcomes may be less than optimal due to the individual's decreased ability to adapt to physical and emotional stressors.

   - The first few days following discharge from an acute care setting can be a period of great vulnerability.
   - Regression from baselines levels of functional ability combined with fatigue and depression, limit rehabilitation potential.

3. Readmission rates have been reported as high as 48%.

4. Evaluation of resources and rehabilitation potential is crucial during the discharge planning process.

5. Statistically, 21% of the elderly do not follow discharge instructions post-discharge.

6. 20% of the discharged elderly claim they do not understand the discharge instructions.

7. 70% of these clients, state that they were not questioned about their ability to care for themselves.

B. Questions to raise during the discharge planning process:

1. What is the functional status of the client and has it been impacted by this current hospitalization?

2. To what degree is the client dependent upon others?

3. Is the client's emotional response to the current situation appropriate, excessive or understated?

4. Did environmental factors such as housing, climate, neighborhood, heat, electricity, fire or safety contribute to the current problem?

5. Is the present problem a new one, or an exacerbation or deterioration of an old one?

6. Is the condition likely to require assistance from family or assistance?

7. Has the client experienced a recent loss; job, financial, home, family member, (spouse)?

8. Does the client have family members or friends who can assist in the recovery process?

9. Are there noted abuses of alcohol, tranquilizers, or misuse of prescription medicines?

10. Are there any social service agencies in place?

11. Does the client have the mental capacity, physical ability, financial means and social support to comply with the recommended treatment plan?

References

1. Kligman, evan M. "Preventive Geriatrics: Basic Principles for Premium Care". Vol 47 #7, July 1992
2. Weinberger, Myron "Hypertension in the Elderly" *Hospital Practice* 5/15/92
3. Ebersole & Hess. *Toward Healthy Aging* (1994)
4. Burgraff, V., Stanley, M. *Nursing the Elderly.* J.B. Lippincott (1989)
5. McDonald, A. "Social Emergencies in the Elderly" *Emergency Medical Clinics of North America.* W.B. Saunders (1990)
6. Hall, M., MacLennon, W.J., Lye, M.P.W. *Medical Care of the Elderly.* John Wiley & Sons Publ.
7. Strange, Gary. "Use of the Emergency Department by Elderly Patients" *Annals of Emergency Medicine* 7/92
8. Hedges, J., Singal, B., Rousseau, E. "Geritric Patient Emergency Visits Part II: Perceptions of Visits by Geriatric and Younger Patients" *Annals of Emergency Medicine*, 21:7 7/92
9. Perez, E.D. "pressure Ulcers; Updated Guidelines for Treatment and Prevention" *Geriatrics* Vol 48,1 1/93

Fig 1. Hall, Michael. "Age Change in Lung Functions" *Medical Care of the Elderly*

Fig 2. Strange, Gary M.D. "Age Distribution for 1990 Emergency Department Visists" *Annals of Emergency Medicine* 21:7 7/92

Fig 3. Singal, Bonita M.D. "Causes of Injury by Patient Group" Annals of Emergency Medicine 21:7 7/92

Fig 4. Singal, M.D., Hedges, M.D. et al. "Reasons for Emergency Department Visits by Patient Group" *Annals of Emergency Medicine* 21:7 7/92

Unit 2 - Chapter 3

Home Health Care for the Elderly Client

The concept of home care began in the late 1700s where vists were made to those who were sick or infirm and generally poor according to religious orders. During the 1800s, there were home care services developed and administered by lay persons utilizing unliscenced, skilled practitioners in the home setting. In the later 1900s, agencies providing care to the sick at home began to appear providing services to the ill by graduate nurses. The Visiting Nurse Association (VNA) was one of the first agencies providing skilled servicealong with being instrumental in developing the fundamentals of home care.

By 1890, there were 21 VNA agencies in the United States. With the advent of World War II, there were fewer physicians available to make home calls, which resulted in the tremendous growth of non-profit home care agencies. By the mid 1960s, it became obvious that with the growing elderly population, the numerous advances in medical tehcnology and society's awareness of and demands for health care, the home care industry would see tremendous growth.

In 1965, with the advent of Medicare and Medicaid, the formation of a federally funded home health program was established. By 1980, Congress had eliminated the pre-hospital requirement and the arbitrary limit on the number of allowable visits a patient may receive, indicating home health care to be a cost effective means of health care delivery and an effective point of entry for a client to receive acute care services.

The development of diagnostic related groups by Medicare in the 1980's has resulted in an every increasing number of home health care agencies filling the gap for patients whoa re discharged from the hospital earlier with higher acuity levels. It is hard to foresee what the next decade will bring to health care, but it is evident to date, that home health care agencies can provide quality and cost effective care to the elderly in their homes, avoiding overutilzation of hospital beds and scarce resources. (NOTE: Medicare is not the only form of reimbursement available to home health agencies, but for this discussion, Medicare will be discussed as the most commonly form used for the geriatric client who seldom pays by other means.)

I. The benefits of home care

A. Acute illness

1. A common point of entry for the elderly client

2. Concerns for the elderly client:

    a. Length of stay

    b. Extent of services

    c. Rehabilitative potential

3. Institutionalization or placement into a longterm care facility is often considered prematurely.

4. Adverse psychosocial effects of acute illness with a proposed institutionalization include:

    a. Emotional distress

    b. Depression.

    c. Disorientation

    d. Agitation

    e. Anxiety

    f. Helplessness

    g. Hopelessness

    h. Despair

B. Effects of institutionalization

1. Families view placement as a tremoundous relief of burden.

2. The elderly client perceives it as abandonment, social isolation and loss of independence.

3. The psychological impact is often underestimated by professionals.

4. The comfort level and equilibrium in a known environment is traded for unknown arena.

5. Loss of a home, pets, and possessions have a profound effect on psychological and physical functioning.

C. Home care after hospital discharge

1. Opportunities exist which can provide for and maintain the elderly individual at home.

2. The home setting provides an arena where a holistic approach can be offered, bringing compassion and individualized care in a familiar environment.

3. Utilization of family and community resources is available in the home setting.

4. Adverse events, such as rehospitalization, nosocomial infections and acute confusional states can be avoided.

5. Home services reduce the cost of care, while eliminating the need for hospital beds.

6. Independence at home with appropriate support systems is, in most cases, the desired outcome.

II. Medicare assessment criteria

A. Client is homebound

1. Client does not have to be bedfast.

2. Client is unable to leave home without a great deal of effort.

3. If client does leave home, it is for a short period of time to seek medical attention:

   a. Private physician appointments

   b. Tests and/or procedures

   c. Radiation and/or chemotherapy

   d. Kidney dialysis

   e. Day care

4. Client requires assistive devices to leave home (cane, walker)

5. Client requires assistance of another person to leave home.

6. Client requires special transportation to leave home:

   a. Wheelchair bound

   b. Bed bound

   c. General weakness

   d. Cardiovascular instability

   e. Visual impairment

   f. Dyspnea

   g. Severe pain

   h. Impaired mobility

   i. Impaired range of motion

   j. Draining wound

B. Client requires intermittent skilled care.

C. Services must be reasonable and necessary. To determine this, the following criteria must be met:
   - Are the skills of the services reasonable and necessary?
   - Will the condition of the client improve in a reasonable and predictable time period?
   - Is home care required to provide a safe and effective plan of care?

III. Goals of home care

The main goal of home care is to successfully manage a client's health care needs at home, a setting which may be more conducive to health restoration and client satisfaction. Health promotion is the key to health restoration, through maintaining or improving the general health of the client.

A. The home health nurse

1. Identifies potential for improvement in physical, psychological and social functioning.

2. Fosters the client's functional abilities

3. Helps to nuture the client's desire to improve self

4. Develops resources to maintain or enhance the client's well-being

5. Serves as an educator

   a. To promote a change in the client's behavior if appropriate

   b. To promote enthusiasm for participation in plan of care

   c. To improve understanding of disease process

   d. To inform of medications, side effects, and importance of regimem

   e. Explains treatments and procedures

   f. Provides written materials to reinforce verbal education

6. Establishes credibility

   a. By developing a rapport with client and caregivers
      - Remembering that the nurse is a guest in the client's home
      - Understanding that the relationship that develops will effect any future efforts to institute or promote health activities

   b. Responds in a way that is non-judgemental

   c. Is supportive as a client advocate

d. Is aware of the family structure and its impact on the achievement of optimal health

B. Health promotion activities

1. Respond to acute and chronic illness, specific to the client's lifestyle

2. Provide individualized health care education

3. Helps the cleint assume more responsiblity for health

4. Client invests in plan of care, focusing on quality of life issues

5. Can avert or delay consequences of acute or chronic illness to prevent further complications

C. Educational programs

1. In the home setting, teaching sessions should be brief and offered frequently

2. Clients need repetition and reinforcement

3. Clients need to verbalize and demonstrate understanding

4. Materials should be at the client's level of understanding, concise and clearly written.

5. The client should have time to process information and respond with questions or concerns.

6. Expected outcomes:

    a. Increased acceptance of responsbility

    b. Development of competency and judgement

    c. Adjustment of behaviors leading to a healthy lifestyle

D. Multidisciplinary team and roles

Care provided by home care agencies is based on a multidisciplinary approach. The therapeutic team in the hospital can be used as a model and adapted to meet the needs of the home-based client. Each discipline is responsible for completing clinical notes which are relevant to each visit.

Professionals who comprise the team:

1. Physicians

    a. Direct plan of care

    b. Signs treatment plan (Medicare Form 485)

    c. Consults with other team members to continually update the plan of care

    d. Review plan of care at least every 62 days

2. Registered nurses

    a. Assesses, plans, implements, evaluates and supervises the client in the home setting

    b. Completes nursing assessment of health needs and evaluates adequacy of home situation to meet the identified needs

    c. Develops plan of care based upon physician's orders and nursing diagnoses

    d. Performs skilled nursing interventions based upon physician orders and nursing care plan

    e. Consults with physician regarding changes in client's condition and renewal of orders as needed

    f. Facilitates client and family teaching

    g. Evaluates client response to plan of care and updates plan of care

    h. Initiates, manages and participates in the discharge planning process

3. Home health aid (usually certified)

    a. Implements and follows prescribed plan of care

    b. Performs a variety of personal care tasks and treatments as directed by nurse or therpaist

    c. Utilizes basic skills to provide client care

d. Utilizes resources within the community for follow-up care

4. Physical therapist

   a. Evaluates and develops plan of care

   b. Instructs and administers physical therapy treatments:
      - Gait and mobility
      - Exercise (strength and range of motion)
      - Biofeedback
      - Ultrasound

   c. Designs therapies which are directed toward relieving pain and/or restoring physiological functions

5. Occupational therapist

   a. Develops therapies which are directed toward restoring function, preventing disability and assisting clients toward maximum ability to function within their capabilities

   b. Evaluates, develops plan of care, instructs and administers treatments

   c. Passive and active exercises, ADL retraining

   d. Muscle retraining

   e. Adaptive devices

6. Speech therapist

   a. Evaluates diagnosis and treatment of communication disorders

   b. Evaluates and diagnoses ability to swallow safely and effectively

7. Clinical nurse specialist

   a. Provides expertise in specialty areas to direct care

   b. Directs staff in developing plan of care

c. Makes consultant visits to clients to evaluate complex client needs and assists in developing plan of care to meet needs

d. Meets/communicates with physican to evaluate plan of care and outcomes

IV. Care and assessment

The plan of care written and directed by the registered nurse, ordered by the physician and integrated along with the multidisciplinary team is best accomplished by use of the nursing process. This plan of care is systematically executed in response to the needs of the client and is closely tailored to the client's own environment. The nursing process includes assessment, development of nursing diagnosis, planning, implementation, intervention, evaluation and continual reassessment. Utilizing these steps during each visit helps to ensure that the client's ever-changing needs are being recognized and met. The client and family should be encouraged and enlisted to participate in this process to ensure their support and cooperation in the recovery period. This process is enhanced by and/or dependent on the family/caregiver taking part in the care and/or health promotion activities which occur during the individual by the home health nurse.

A. The nursing process applied

Assessment (collection of data, developing plan of care, client problem/needs identified, identified areas which lack sufficient knowledge to manage health care needs)

1. Physical assessment

    a. Integumentary

    - Assess for temperature, moisture, diaphoresis, color, rash, itching, bruising, pressure areas, incisions, oral mucosa, capillary refill

    b. Musculoskeletal

    - Assess for falls, weakness, paralysis, assistive devices, gait, balance, range of motion

    c. Neurologic

    - Assess for dizziness, headaches, tremors, seizures, pupil response

d. Cardiopulmonary
   - Assess for arrhythmias, palpiataitons, chest pain, shortness of breath, crepitus, rales, rhonchi, wheezing, breath sounds, cough, sputum, cyanosis, pedal pulses, edema
e. Gastrointestinal system
   - Assess for appetite, nutrition and hydration, nausea, vomiting, pain, bleeding, flatus, bowel habits, bowel sounds, enteral nutrition, use of dietary supplements
f. Genitourinary
   - Assess for dysuria, frequency, hematuria, retention, incontinence, use of catheters, burning or paing, ostomy, perineal area, discharge, sexual dysfunction
g. EENT
   - Assess for dysphagia, aphasia, hearing loss, pain, drainage, redness, visual impairment
h. Endocrine
   - Assess blood glucose levels, thyroid function
i. Pain
   - Assess location, severity, effective treatments, medications, effects on ADLs
j. Emotional presentation
   - Assess for level of alertness, orientation, mood, memory and cooperation

B. Ability to Perform Activities of Daily Living
   1. Eating, drinking
   2. Dressing, grooming
   3. Toileting, hygiene
   4. Ambulation, transferring self

C. Ability to perform instrumental activities of daily living
   1. Preparing meals, snacks
   2. Housekeeping

3. Laundry
4. Handling finances
5. Use of telephone

D. Safety of the environment
   1. Safety of the neighborhood (high crime area)
   2. Structural safety and barriers to independent functioning
   3. Amount of time caregiver is present
   4. Status of utilities
   5. Emergency plans
   6. Electrical safety
   7. Pets, pests
   8. Appropriate water temperature
   9. Basic safety of appliances, (i.e. stove, heaters)

E. Past medical history
   1. Hospitalizations within last 6 months
   2. Allergies
   3. Integumentary disorders (herpes simplex, herpes zoster, pressure areas, skin tears)
   4. EENT disorders (cataracts, cancers, macular degeneration, glaucoma)
   5. Cardiopulmonary impairment (MI, CHF, CABG, HTN, COPD, asthma, cancers, pneumonia)
   6. Gastrointestinal disorders (ulcers, ostomy, hepatitis, hernia, cancer)
   7. Musculoskeletal disorders (fractures, arthritis, amputee)
   8. Neurologic disorders (CVA, TIA, paralysis, cancers, Parkinson's, neuropathy)
   9. Endocrine disorders (diabetes, thyroid, tumor, cancers)

10. Genitourinary/gynecologic disorders (UTI, incontinence, ostomy, venereal disease, discharge)
11. Mental/emotional disorders (depression, psychosis, anxiety, behavior disorders, dementia, schizophrenia, bipolar affective disorder)

F. Demographics
   1. Name, age, birthdate
   2. Address, phone number,
   3. Primary physician, address, phone
   4. Primary caregiver, address, phone
   5. Emergency contacts, address, phone
   6. Other agencies involved
   7. Medical equipment supplier
   8. Pharmacy

G. Family/caregiver ability/willingness to participate
   1. Reliability of caregiver as well as ability to understand treatments, protocols
   2. Family resistance may indicate ambivalence
   3. Family's fear of being unable to cope with care issues may be dispelled when professional help is available

H. Nursing diagnosis

   Problems and specific knowledge deficits are identified based on information gleaned from the initial nursing assessment. The nursing diagnosis should be determined after a system's review:
   1. Alteration in urinary output related to . . . .
   2. Alteration in cardiac output related to . . . .
   3. Knowledge deficit related to diabetic care management . . .
   4. Electrolyte imbalance related to . . . .
   5. Alteration in cardiovascular status related to . . . .

6. Alteration in pulmonary status related to . . . .

7. Self-care deficit

8. Altered verbal communication related to . . . .

9. Ineffective individual coping

10. Inability of family to cope with care issues . . . .

11. Alteration in mobility related to . . . .

12. Potential for falls secondary to orthostatic hypotension

I. Planning

This phase includes setting goals and objectives to accomplish the plan of care. Goals are action oriented, time limited and must be tailored to the individual client and family to produce successful interventions. The client and family are integral in this phase of the nursing process because the burden of meeting goals rests on their shoulders. The family is responsible for implementing interventions to meet the established goals.

Examples:

1. Knowledge deficit related to diabetic care, management and goals;

    a. Blood sugars consistently below 200 at time of discharge

    b. Client/caregiver to verbalize and demonstrate when appropriate ability to manage diabetic care by the time of disharge

    c. Early detection of unstable blood sugars during home health coverage period

2. Alteration in cardiovascular status related to hypertension goals;

    a. Controlled hypertension-diastolic of 90mm/Hg or below by time of discharge

    b. Early detection of unstable BP during home care coverage period

c. Client/caregiver able to manage diet and medicaton regime

   d. Client/caregiver to verbalize reportable changes in health status during coverage period

   e. Client/caregiver to verbalize understanding of medication purpose and side effects during coverage period.

   f. Client/caregiver able to demonstrate ability to monitor own BP by time of discharge

J. Interventions

   Interventions are based on the plan of care which includes the treatments, procedures or educational component necessary to enhance the client and family's knowledge base.

   Working along side the client and family gives the professional caregiver the opportunity to not only teach from experience, but also by example those methods necessary to prevent exacerbation and to promote healing. The selected interventions should be achievable, reasonable and meaningful for optimal health.

   Example:

   1. Knowledge deficit related to diabetic care management Interventions;

      a. Assess client/caregiver knowledge of diabetes and its implications

      b. Assess client/caregiver knowledge of diabetes care issues, short and long term

      c. Instruct client/caregiver according to individualized needs

      d. Inform of signs and symptoms of hyper- and hypoglycemia and appropriate measures

      e. Instruct regarding insulin administration

      f. Instruct purpose, side effects of insulin or oral hypoglycemic products

      g. Instruct on need for good foot care

      h. Inform client/family of emergency procedures

i. Educate regarding diet regulations

j. Educate regarding use of home glucose monitoring system

2. Alteration in cardiovascular status related to hypertension; Interventions:

a. Assess cardiovascular status/vital signs

b. Assess side effects/benefits of medications

c. Instruct client/caregiver of medication regimen

d. Assess/instruct knowledge of dietary restrictions

e. Instruct regarding reportable changes in blood pressure

f. Instruct regarding using of home BP monitoring equipment

g. Instruct client/caregiver in the use of emergency procedures

K. Evaluation

This procss, like all others, requires ongoing evalutaion of the client's progress. It is possible to measure outcomes by asking the following questions;

1. Have goals and objectives been met?

2. What has the client/caregiver learned to help prevent further exacerbations or decline?

3. Has the client made any necessary behavior changes?

4. Has the client/caregiver gained knowledge needed to control the disease process?

5. Has the client/caregiver learned to manage care?

6. Can the client continue to be managed at home?

7. What is the client/caregiver's response to the home care environment?

The Outline Series - Geriatric Nursing -- 235

- L. Documentation
    1. Must be precise, reflecting the day-to-day status of the client.
    2. Reflects and validates the need for services and care in the home
    3. Justifies reimbursement and provides evidence of services
    4. Records changes in condition as evidenced by telephone conversations and extra visits
    5. Includes the identified problems, the goals and interventions, all physician orders, home health aid care plans, the interdisplinary team's progress notes, and current medication records

V. Ethical issues

- A. Ethical issues in home care must also deal with the acuity and the urgency of services being provided.

    Issues include:
    1. Justification for reimbursement
    2. Life sustaining methods
    3. End of life choices
    4. Willingess of caregiver to carry out treatment
- B. Suitability and availability of services can raise ethical questions:
    1. Can needed treatments be provided to client?
    2. Can treatments be performed safely in the environment?
    3. Is this environment the appropriate setting for treatments?
    4. Is the health care team qualified to carry out the prescribed treatments?
    5. Is client/caregiver compliant with treatment?
    6. Are there issues of ambivalence between client and caregiver?

7. Should services be continued if client/caregiver displays non-compliance?

8. Is referral to a community abuse/neglect hotline appropriate?

C. Steps in solving ethical questions:

1. Identify problem (rely on facts, not opinion)

2. Gather information which describes the situation

3. Determine course of action

4. Think problem through

5. Decide on the best approach to the problem

6. Carry out actions to solve the problem

D. Responsibility of the nurse

1. Facilitates communication between client, physician and health care team

2. Considers the values, ideals, morals, principals and life experiences which affect the situation.

3. Keeps the client's best interest in mind during the decision making process

4. Shows constant support, respect and concern for client and family.

5. Must possess knowledge of complex technology, skills and sound clinical judgement to manage severely ill clients.

VI. Caregivers

A. Family responsibility

1. Encouraged and supported by government policy

2. The spouse is usually the main caregiver; in circumstances where there is not a spouse available, a daughter takes on responsibility.

3. Without family caregivers, many elderly with functional disabilities would be institutionalized.

4. Requires 24 hr. vigilance and adjustment of schedules at home to accomodate the infirmed.

5. Physical demands of caregiving can be devastating to the home environment and family life.

6. Caregivers should be viewed as hidden patients, who are physically and emotionally drained from the demands of a dependent parent or loved one.

7. Encompasses not only the physical care required, but also the overall responsibility for that individual, until recovery is complete

B. Support systems

1. Intervention to relieve the plight of caregivers is needed to avoid the strains of isolation and loss of independence while providing 24 hr. care.

2. Effective management of care issues as well as one's personal life is essential.

3. Health care professionals can observe the caregiver in the environment to assess functioning, physical limitations and emotional stress.

4. Support for the caregiver should be explored in terms of additional family members, respite services, community resources and church affiliations.

C. Hospice

Hospice clients are some of the most critically ill in the health care system. Clients have physical, emotional, social and spiritual concerns.

1. Hospice benefits for the terminally client have been available through the Medicare program since 1983. Benefit periods vary, depending on the needs of the individual.

2. Provides an interdisciplinary team consisting of primary physicians, nurses and social workers to serve the needs of the client and family.

3. Requirements for hospice:
   - Order from physician
   - Client will succumb within 6 month time frame

- No extraordinary measures to be performed
- Client and family to agree to hospice format

4. Philosophy includes:

    a. Providing care not cure

    b. Keeping the client in a home-like setting

    c. Providing care by the interdisciplinary team

    d. Providing education and comfort with the goal of helping the client and family bridge the transition from life to death as peaceful as possible.

5. Care is designed to meet the needs of the client and family, improving quality of life, not extending it.

6. Efforts are made to help the client live as fully and comfortably as possible, realizing that the dying process requires assistance.

7. Hospice caregivers are sensitive to the demands of the client through listening, being supportive and providing assistance to ease the burden.

CONCLUSION

As the home health industry evolves, the care issues will be shaped by the acuity levels of clients in the home setting, the use of increased medical technology outside of the hospital, ever-changing reimbursement systems and changes in the nature of problems seen in the home. There now exists a wider variety of services being offered in the home setting to meet the growing demands in this area. All agencies will need to offer services on an expanded level to remain competitive in the service market. Areas of growth and potential for greater share of the market include home IV therapy, private duty and homemaker services.

Unit 3

The Elderly Individual: Legal And Social Issues

Unit 3 - Chapter 1

Politics of Aging

I. Introduction

There are many reasons why legislators are paying increasing attention to the elderly:

A. Financial concerns

1. The immediate concerns are for protection from inflation for those on fixed incomes.

2. Rising costs for goods and services in addition to depletion of pensions and assets pose a frightening dilemma for the elderly as well as those who care for them.

B. Economic effects

1. The effect on the increasing numbers of families caught in the sandwich generation is having a major impact not only on the basic family unit but also on the economic climate of our country.

2. Never before have there been the number of children caring for parents and their own children.

3. The burden of employment, elder care issues, and the demands of a growing family place today's boomers at risk for great physical, psychological and financial stress. The elderly-support ratio which is a figure representing the number of working individuals compared to those who are retired is changing significantly. ZPG (Zero Population Growth) of the '70's is now becoming painfully evident.

4. The ratio of caregivers to careneeders is disproportionate and predictions are that this ratio will continue to decline.

5. The cost of getting well and staying well for ourselves and our aging parents is astronomical.

6. Shrinking Social Security funds, cut-backs in government-supplemented insurance programs and private plans, and basic health care cost becomes less affordable every year.

II. Policies

A. Health policies for the elderly

1. Introduction of disability insurance 1956
2. Medicare developed 1965
3. Cost or living benefit 1972
4. OBRA (Omnibus Reconciliation Act) 1987
5. Medicaid laws changed to protect assets 1988
6. Yearly reimbursement limits for Medicare abolished 1990
7. Family Support Act 1991

B. Civil rights for the elderly

1. The 1960's brought about a national cry for the rights of the individual.

2. Minorities including ethnic, cultural and religious groups as well as those impaired because of disease, congenital defects or age were the victims of blatant discrimination.

3. The Civil Rights Movement awakened an awareness in all of us of the inequities in our society.

4. Political activists worked valiantly for decades to bring about change and fairness for all, regardless of race, creed or physical ability.
   - Access to public accomodations, employment and educational opportunities was achieved.

5. Those in power realized that all people included those those at the far end of the spectrum; those who had contributed millions of hours in the labor force, had brought us through two World Wars and assured that our country would always be a land of freedom.

6. The political activity of this country was driven by the need for equity and justice and fear of repercussion for exclusivity.

7. The passage of the Older American's Act (1965) and the Senior Citizen's Bill of Rights, as well as senior activists like Claude Pepper and Maggie Kuhn guaranteed a chance for better quality of life, free from devastating poverty and powerlessness.

III. Medicare

A two-part federally funded health insurance plan to help recipients afford medical expenses. Eligibility is based on several factors:

- The individual must be 65 or older and qualify for Social Security benefits
- Disability with Social Security benefits for two years for any age group
- Recipient of kidney dialysis or waiting for a kidney transplant

It is governed by the Health Care Finance Adminstration (HCFA) hich contracts with private insurance companies (intermediaries) to administer policies.

A. The original Medicare plans included:

1. Coverage for those over the age of 65 as well as the physically and mentally challenged was imperative.

2. A design to meet the acute health care needs, without regard for chronic or long term care, dealing with medical services directed toward the disease, rather than the resolution of the consequences of the disabling illness

3. There were no provisions for care that was other than reasonable and necessary, (psychologic or non-medical services).

B. The role of the intermediaries

1. Process medical claims

2. Make interim payments

3. Review cost reports

C. Types of coverage

The scope of service varies greatly from one to another, based upon individual interpretation of the Medicare guidelines. Because this is one of the entitlement programs, it is at risk for drastic changes based on the economy and political climate.

1. Medicare Type A; also known as hospital coverage

    Necessary services include:
    - Hospitalization
    - Nursing and related services
    - Operating and recovery room costs
    - Diagnostic and therapeutic services, such as rehabilitation

    One of the limitations is the lack of coverage for preventive care.

    a. Care which can only be provided in a Skilled Nursing Facility (SNF) is covered when the person requires skilled nursing or rehabilitation which can only be provided under the supervision of a professional or technical personnel
        - The patient's condition is often the deciding factor in determining whether the service is skilled or non-skilled as opposed to the diagnosis.

        Examples of skilled services include;
        - Management and evaluation of a patient care plan
        - Observation and assessment of the patient's condtion
        - Teaching and training activities
        - Direct skilled procedures to treat Stage III or IV pressure ulcers on the trunk of the body
        - Gastric tube feedings

        Examples of non-skilled services include:
        - Administration of routine oral medications eyedrops and ointments
        - General maintenance care of colostomy and ileostomy
        - Routine services to maintain satisfactory functioning indwelling bladder catheters

- Changes of dressings for non-infected post-operative or chronic conditions
- Prophylactic and palliative skin care, including bathing and application of creams or treatment of minor skin problems
- Routine care of the incontinent patient, including use of diapers and protective sheets
- General maintenenace care in connection with a plaster cast
- Routine care in connection with braces and similar devices
- Use of heat as a palliative and comfort measures, such as whirlpool or heat pack
- Routine administration of oxygen after a regimen of therapy has been established
- Assistance in dressing, eating and going to the toilet
- Periodic turning and positioning in bed
- General supervision of exercises which have been taught to the patient and the performance of repetitious exercises that do not require skilled rehabilitation personnel for their performance

b. The person requires these services on a daily basis

c. Considering economy and efficiency, the skilled services can be provided only on an inpatient basis in a SNF

d. The services must be provided pursuant to a physician's order and be reasonable and necessary for the treatment of the patient's illness or injury.

e. The service must be reasonable in terms of duration and quantity.

f. If full or partial recovery is not a possibility the skilled service may be covered if it is to prevent deterioration or to maintain current functional ability.
- Complications which may occur without skilled services:
1) contractures

2) loss of muscle tone

3) pressure ulcers

4) immobility

2. Skilled nursing facility services which are covered:

   a. Semi-private accomodations

   b. Medical supplies and oxygen

   c. Drugs both prescription and non-prescription

   d. Physical therapy

   e. Occupatioinal therapy

   f. Speech therapy

   g. Respiratory therapy

   h. Lab and X-Ray

3. Medicare Type B, also known as supplemental medical insurance is an optional plan which covers physician and outpatient services and others which may not be covered by Type A including specific nursing home services and outpatient rehabilitation and certain care within community and mental health centers. Type B is automatically taken out of the monthly Social Security check, unless otherwise specified.

   Type B criteria:

   - Existing eligibility for Part A and/or pay a monthly premium of approximately $45.00/mo.

   - Part B is optional and may be purchased without Part A

4. In a skilled nursing facility the following services are covered:

   - Speech, physical and occupational therapy

   - Physician's services and supplies

   - Diagnositc lab and radiology services

   - Surgical dressings and supplies

   - Durable medical equipment (oxygen, wheel- chairs, hospital beds)

   - Ambulance services

- Prosthetic devices
- Braces, splints, trusses and artificial limbs
- Pneumococcal/Influenza and Hepatitis B Vaccine
- Portable dialysis systems
- Outpatient dialysis

5. For the elderly individual living in the community:
   - Rural health clinic services
   - Comprehensive outpatient rehabilitation services
   - Ambulatory surgical facility services
   - Health maintenance organization services
   - Hospital outpatient services

6. When the services covered under Part A are exhausted, Part B can be applied.

7. Coverage is more extensive if the services are provided in the home, and when the care is considered to be reasonable, necessary and is directed by a physician order.

8. The provider of service must be Medicare approved

9. The fee structure requires the beneficiary to the required co-payment and pay 20% of the service. Medicare covers the remaining 80%.

IV. Medicaid

A program established to provide medical care for the low-income, often-unemployed individual. Coverage for the elderly includes hospitalization and long-term care with specific spend down specifications, or reduce assets.

A. It may cover specific physician office visits, dental visits, prescription drugs, emergency ambulance service, out patient. hospital services, lab and radiology serivces, optometric services, periodic diagnostic and screening services, and home health services.

B. Institutions may limit number of Medicaid beds available.

C. Eligibility requires the individual to be:
- Current recipient of funds from a state agency, i.e. General Relief, State supplemental payments.
- Disabled due to visual impairment with a gross monthly income of less than approximately $400.00/mo for an individual or $600.00/mo for a couple.

D. Some drugs and services require prior authorization.

V. Current issues

The legislative power of the elderly lies with those who have the interest, energy and endurance to work in a system that inherently discriminates against minority groups.

A. Today's aging population
1. There are millions of poor, socioeconomically deprived and impaired elderly who do not vote, are usually not aware of the issues and gain very little from the process.
2. Seniors who have the time to become politically involved, are usually concerned with those policies which affect them specifically:
   - Social Security not Supplemental Security Income
   - Medicare not Medicaid

B. Health care reform

Though millions of elderly live in fear that their health care coverage will be inadequate, many are optimistic about the prospect for change.

1. Federal plans
   a. Current leglislative issues are meeting with universal controversy, despite the need for global revisions.
   b. Universal coverage is defined as a plan which would provde a health care umbrella, with employers assuming more of the expenses cooperating with health alliances to make policies more affordable.
   c. Medicare coverage would see limited changes, with the hope of additional choices regarding physicians and other options.

d. Medical providers would reorganize into managed care networks to treat people more efficiently.

 2. Current plans must include:

   a. Availability to persons of all ages, races and incomes with protection for those the lowest socioeconomic strata

   b. Provision of benefits to persons with cognitive and mental impairments as well as physical disabiliites

   c. Emphasis on home and community services which are culturally and economically feasible

   d. Flexibility to meet individual needs as defined by a prescribed plan of care

   e. Provision of consumer choices for services providers

   f. Financial appropriations across generations and with guidelines for meaningful cost containment

   g. Consideration for the most efficient long term care programs and a framework for a full coverage social insurance plan

   h. Provision for research for those illnesses which cost society millions of dollars annually in treatments, acute and long term care which provide

VI. Alzheimer's Disease

 A. The current facts

  1. One of the greatest emerging health concerns of this century, affecting every sector of our older society

  2. It is the third leading cause of death in the elderly

  3. Currently 4 million Americans with this insidious disease

   - Predicitions are that this number will triple in the next 50 years.

4. AD affects global functioning, causing physical and cognitive deterioration, robbing the individual of the ability to think, live independently and perform normal daily activities

B. Health care's system response to AD
  1. There has been an overwhelming response to the educational, psychological and emotional needs of the AD patient and family members.
  2. Financial support, as well as long term care benefits for these patients as well as others with chronic disease are sorely lacking.
  3. Hence, the majority of care is provided in the home or in residential care settings.
  4. The cost rises annually, reaching approximately $100 billion per year.
  5. Families are absorbing the majority of these costs.
  6. Medicare and most private health plans do not cover the cost of care.
  7. Medicaid is usually a last resort when a family has exhausted their own resources and are ready to seek long term care placement.
  8. Further development of community and home care services could eliminate or reduce many of the hospitalizations which result from acute episodes of illness for the AD patient, saving millions of dollars per year.

C. The caregivers
  1. The burden upon those who provide care is physically, financially, and emotionally draining.
  2. Care is usually provided by the spouse an individual who is also elderly, with emotional and health care needs as well.
  3. Immediate family members, usually adult children also assume responsibility for care, struggling with their own families, careers and financial concerns.

4. Statistically, the caregiver of the AD victim will begin to lose physical and psychological well-being in more than 50% of the cases over a period of time.

D. The needs

1. Support for community and home based services is essential, allowing family to remain as primary caregivers, providing individualized and personalized attention.

2. Mechanisms which provide for financial support in dealing with the long term care issues would contain escalating health care costs.

3. Research funding to find the cure as well as clinical markers for early detection

4. Support for the Family Caregiver Support Act, which would provide a program of respite services to families caring for the AD patients and others who require constant care and superivison

5. Continued development of Alzheimer's Disease Centers which aid in the identification of culturally deprived areas, serving urban, rural and minority communities.

VII. Family Support Act of 1992

A. Definition

Formulated to assist caregivers whose role has been misunderstood.

1. Caregivers under this plan are defined as those who give assistance with at least 3 out of 5 activities of daily living for the individual who is either incompetent or cognitively impaired.

2. Places demands on the emloyers of caregivers who remain in the work force to allow for leave of absences, time, and flexibility in the work environment.

B. Guidelines

1. Allows for paid and unpaid family leave which fits criteria

2. In some communities, provides on-site elder care services which offer resources and support to the caregiver

VIII. Adult protective services

A. Definition

A system of preventive, suportive and surrogate services for the elderly, living in the community to enable them to maintain independent living and avoid abuse and exploitation.

Services may be in one of two categories:

1. Coordinated delivery of care

2. Actual or potential authority to provide substitute decision-making.

B. Funded through Title 20 of the Socialy Security Act and Title 3 of the Older Americans' Act

IX. American Association of Retired Persons (AARP)

A. Who are the AARP?

1. The largest organization of Americans over the age of 50

2. Approximately 30 million members nationwide

3. Originally organized as a nonprofit corporation for the purpose of promoting the interest of older persons.

B. Functions of the AARP

1. Legislative advocate at the state and federal level

2. Political concerns include:
   - Social Security
   - Medicare
   - Long-term care issues
   - Health care
   - Housing needs
   - Age discrimination
   - Elderly abuse
   - Crime prevention

C. Benefits of membership
   1. Group health insurance program
   2. Meciare supplement plans
   3. Non-profit mail-order pharmacy
   4. Auto-homeowner insurance programs
   5. Amoco Motor Club-emergency road service
   6. Travel service
   7. Investment service
   8. Servcie providers and discounts available to members at participating lodging, airlines, sight-seeing and car rental companies
   9. Federal credit union
D. Local and community programs
   1. Driver education . . . "55 Alive/Mature Driving"
   2. Crime prevention programs that teach preventive measures
   3. Elder health
   4. Health fairs
   5. Medication awareness/Educational programs
   6. IRS-trained AARP volunteers
   7. Volunteer talent bank
   8. Medicare-Medicaid assistance in dealing with insurance complexities
   9. Safety and injury prevention
   10. Widowed persons service
   11. Women's health programs

X. The Gray Panthers

A. Definition;

A social activist organization with members of all ages to create a society with dignity from birth to death. The organization was founded in 1970 by Maggie Kuhn when she was forced to retire along with 5 friends at the age of 65.

B. Accomplishments

1. Led the sucessful fight against forced retirement at age 65

2. Exposed shocking nursing home abuse that led to convictions and tough new laws

3. Helped convince FDA to monitor and regulate the hearing aid industry for fraudulent practices

4. Mobilized hundreds of thousands to fight and beat many plans to increase military spending which would have detracted from the Medicare and Medicaid entitlement programs.

XI. National Council of Senior Citizens

A. NSCS is an advocacy organization, dedicated to the belief that America's elderly are worthy of the best that this nation can give.

B. Purpose of the NSCS

1. Preserve Social Security

2. Protect Medicare and Medicaid

3. Expand job opportunities for people over the the age of 50

4. Protect senior centers, nurtional programs and other elder programs which aid older Americans.

C. The local chapters

1. Prevent doctors from charging more than the Medicare-assigned rates

2. Maintain accurate information regarding nursing home access and appropriate regulations

3. Monitor Lifeline utility rates for the elderly

4. Keep prescription rates for Medicare patients within reason

5. Build affordable senior housing

6. Sponsor local programs to make health care more affordable

7. Provide adult care to help older people remain in their homes

XII. National Council on Aging, Inc.

A. Defined: The nation's leading resource for professionals serving the aged. Established in 1950, NCOA has provided training, technical assistance and information to those dedicated to the care of the older person.

B. Political issues:

1. Supports long term care programs

2. Supports social service agencies

3. Works for better housing, improved housing and health benefits

C. Organizations which interface with NCOA

1. NAOWES . . . National Association of Older Workers' Employment Services

2. NCRA . . . National Center on Rural Aging

3. NIAD . . . Naitonal Institute on Adult Daycare

4. NICLC . . . National Institute on Community-based Long Term Care

5. NISC . . . National Institute on Senior Centers

6. NISH . . . National Institute on Senior Housing

7. NVOILA . . . Naitonal Voluntary Organizations for Independent Living for the Aging

8. NIHPOA . . . National Institute on Health Promotion for Older Adults.

XIII. The Omnibus Reconciliation Act of 1987 (OBRA)

Philosophy states that "Each resident must receive and the facility must provide the necessary care and services to attain or maintain the highest practicable physical, mental and psychosocial well-being. The facility must promote care for residents in a manner and in an environment that maintains or enhances each resident's dignity and respect in full recognition of his or her individuality."

A. Defined: A program developed to improve the lives of nursing home residents.

1. Directs care toward meeting psychosocial needs, preventing deterioration and recognizing risk factors.

2. Changes in nursing home policy and procedures have been enacted to lessen the incidence of abuse and neglect.

B. Regulations which have accomplished the elimination of many problematic areas:

1. Use of restraints, both physical and chemical

2. Mandated professional social services in facilities with 120 beds or more

3. Certification and continuing educatioin for nursing assistants

4. Penalties for abuse

5. Documentation of issues related to resident's rights

XIV. Older Americans' Act (OAA)

A. Philosophy: To serve those elderly in the greatest social and economic need, giving particular attention to low income minority individuals and providing services and programs that assist in maintaining independence as well as dignity

1. Federal OAA has established certain programs that must be implemented by the states, with the assistance of federal funds.

2. States establish their own Department of Aging to implement the provisions of the OAA and act as a unifying force for services to seniors.

3. States also participate in providing additional funds and entitlement programs for seniors.

4. Area Agencies on Aging operate as local units to work with other private non-profit agencies to implement other desired programs.

B. Division by titles and operations:

1. TITLE I...Declaration of Objective

Sets the broad national social policy objectives toward improving the lives of older Americans including:

a. Adequate income for retirement

b. Optimum physical and mental health

c. Suitable housing designed and located to meet special needs

d. Full restorative servcies for those who require institutionalization including a comprehensive array of community-based long term care services

e. Opportunity for employment without age discrimination

f. Retirement in health, honor and dignity

g. Pursuit of civic, cultural, education, training and recreational opportunities

h. Efficient community services with emphasis on maintaining a continuum of care for the vulnerable elderly

i. Benefits from research designed to sustain and improve health and happiness

j. Freedom for older persons to plan and manage their lives, participate in the planning and operation of services designed for their benefit, and protection against abuse, neglect and exploitation

2. TITLE II Administration on Aging

    Established within the Department of Health and Human Services to administer the program. Also established the Federal Council on Aging, an advisory body to the president and to Congress.

3. TITLE III

    Grants for state and community programs on Aging. Title III provides grants to state and area agencies on aging to develop supportive and nutritional services, to act as advocates on behalf of programs for older persons, and to coordinate programs for the elderly. The programs is intended to form a network to link AOA, state and area agencies on aging as well as public and private agencies, social and nutrional providers.

4. TITLE III B...Supportive Services

    a. Adult day healthcare

    b. Alzheimer's day care centers

    c. Assistance to older persons with special needs

    d. Brown Bag Network Program

    e. Elder abuse prevention activities

    f. Foster grandparent program

    g. Health education and promotion services

    h. Health insurance counseling and advocacy program

    i. Information and referral

    j. In-home services

    k. Legal assistance

    l. Linkages

    m. Long-term care ombudsman service

    n. Outreach activities

    o. Respite care

p. Senior centers

q. Senior discount program

r. Transportation

5. TITLE IV...Training, Research and Discretionary Projects and Programs

Assists in support and development of the following programs:

a. Community based long-term care

b. Adult literacy

c. Alzheimer's disease support services

d. Training for those employed in the field of aging

e. Studies in the area of health care, housing, social services, retirement roles, and the needs of low-income and minority older persons.

f. Funding to support innovative approaches to provide services under this Act.

6. TITLT V...Senior Community Service Employment Program

- Designed to provide funds to subsidize, foster and promote useful part-time opportunities in community service employment for the unemployed, low-income persons 55 years or older. Also to assist in the transition of enrollees to private or other unsubsidized employment

7. TITLE VI...Grants to Native Americans

- Authorizes funds for social and nutritional services awarded directly to tribal organizations of older Indians and native Hawaiians.[1]

C. Older Women's League

- (OWL) National grassroots membership organization which focuses on the needs and concerns of women as they age. Its goals include support for members to achieve economic and social equity and to improve the image and status of older women.

D. MCFU
- Medicaid Fraud Control Units provide investigations and prosecution of abuse and neglect cases involving health care facility residents

XV. Government agencies

A. The role of government agencies for the elderly;
1. To meet the demands of this population with a growing number of services necessaryb and an ever-shrinking budget.
2. To identify those in need of public assistance
3. To help those who are finding new difficulties in caring for themselves, maintaining current levels of independence and planning for anticipated losses.
4. To support those who are providing care by offering respite services and financial assistance.

B. Community programs funded through governmental support
1. Senior fairs offer a variety of services through a 'vendor' approach. Attendees can learn about products, programs and organizations designed especiallly for the senior market. In addition, the opportunity to find out about social and community organizations is available.
2. Older resident programs offer information and referral services, crime prevention, help services for filing taxes, medical claim forms and legal advice. There are also opportunities for those who wish to volunteer, may be homebound or are looking for employment.

XVI. The Political Future of Health Care

Historically, policy makers have overlooked para-professional work force issues while focusing on rising costs, long term care issues and the necessary expenditures to meet the demands. The discussions regarding the cost of health care and the possibilities which exist about its rationalization have yet to produce solid solutions. The committment to provide health care to all and the limitations imposed by the resources available to fund this care demands a systematic and regulated approach to the delivery of these services.

A. Ethical and medical policy guidelines:

1. Limit specific types of care to particular individuals. (extraordinary measures for those who are old old or who may be severely debilitated are not considered to be reasonable and just.)

2. The National Service Program and any programs developed to expand employment opportunities should include employment, training, and career opportunities in long term care.

B. Financial policies

Place budgetary restrictions on the total amount of care, leaving the remainder of expenses to private payers.

1. Spousal impoverishment limitations should be readdressed, allowing the remaining older adult to preserve their own environment and sense of security.

2. Hardship exemptions and estate recovery requirements should be established

3. Long term care expenses should be treated by the Internal Revenue Service as medical expenses.

4. Congress should continue existing programs that would provide the base for effective implementation of long term care under Health Care Reform.

5. Programs authorized by TITLE III of the Older Americans' Act to provide services for frail older persons should be fully funded.

C. Citizen-driven policies

Policies which encourage patient input into the choices regarding the extent of medical care one wishes to receive and the alternatives available, (The Self Determination Act)

1. Uniform national standards for private long term care insurance should be enacted along with strong consumer protection laws.

2. Department of Housing and Urban Development should ensure that supportive services designed to allow frail older persons to remain in their own homes or otherwise age in place, including appropriate services for persons with dementia. (Alzheimer's Public Policy, Inc.)

3. Specialized training for caregivers in the home as well as in the institutional setting is essential.

4. The need for creation and development of such programs is obvious.

D. The political economy

1. There is an existing strong influence from policy makers and legislators on the health care community

    - This population includes those working in hospitals, long-term care settings, and the home health environment. Typically, the majority of these care providers are female, whose careers depend on a sense of security within the health care setting.

2. Financial constraints, dictated by the political economy, govern long-term care workers wages, benefits and job descriptions.

3. The need for profit maximization, rationalization of resources and organiational changes creates conflict among client needs, labor's efforts and corportate policies.

4. The medical model and the cost of providing care are directed currently under the regulations of Medicare and Medicaid.

XVII. Recommendations for Quality Health Care in the 21st Century

A. The increasing demand on health care providers

1. The growing number of individuals reaching their eight, ninth and tenth decade is ever-increasing.

2. Age brings about changes, often decline in functional, cognitive and emotional abilities.

3. The shortage of well-trained, qualified direct-care workers may be see as the sleeping giant of this century.

4. Continued efforts to enhance the front line workers' ability to become more effective and efficient in the provision of care is critical.

5. Early detection of disease as well as regular screening for sings of functinal, physical and and cognitive impairment lowers the risk for serious complications.

B. The expectations of the client

1. The elderly client is most affected by the strict regulations and limitations imposed by public policy.

2. The needs of the client evolve in the second fifty years, requiring further reimbursement and research in the field of preventive medicine, lower costs for medications and physician office visits, and protection for spouses during times of catastrophic illness.

3. Palliative measures which avoid aggressive and traumatic interventions are often preferred by the elderly client.

4. The provision of comfort measures and the recognition of quality of life issues can only be provided by those who understand the aging process and have a compassionate view of the client's place in the life cycle.

C. Research issues

1. Funding which explores the aging process and related diseases as well as the cost-effectiveness of treatments is imperative.

   - The cost of health care interventions to treat disease and debilitation is astronomical compared to that which could maintain health and abilities.

2. The need for further studies into the causes and treatments for those with dementing illness is critical as one recognizes the added burden these individuals place on the health care team.

   - The individual with dementia who also becomes acutely ill requires additional resources, time and consultation during hospitalization, not to mention the added risk issues involved in an institutional setting.

3. The benefits of rehabilitative therapy for the elderly are being recognized as a means of maintaining or restructuring functional abilities which keeps the dependency ratio at lower levels.
   - Studies have shown that walkers, wheelchairs and canes are being replaced or eliminated for many individuals who are benefitting from weight training and routine exercises which improve muscle strenght and capacity.
4. The study of falls in the elderly have revealed a complexity of issues which cost society billions of dollars annually. Research which leads to further investigation of those at risk for falls and preventive measures is essential.

CONCLUSION

In conclusion, the twenty-first century is approaching rapidly and the projected numbers of elderly and the surrounding issues will be overwhelmingly challenging. The mean age of the population will be fifty years, with more than 20% over the age of 65. The growth of this segment and the resultant economic issues will force a restructuring of the policital and medical society in our country. The pressure on society to provide extensive services, policies for this groups will cause reorganization at every level. Age-based restrictions as well as discriminatory practices will become obsolete and functional ability will re-define personal potential and purpose.

References

Cheney, W., Diehm, W.J., and Seeley, F.E. *The Second Fifty Years*. Paragon House Publishers, New York, NY (1992)

Alzheimer's Association. National Public Policy Program. Chicao, IL

Day, C.I. *What Older Americans Think*. Princeton University Press, Princeton, NJ (1990)

Minkler, M. and Estes, C. *Critical Persepctives on Aging: The Political and Morale Economy of Growing Old*. Baywood Publishing Co. Amityville, NY (1991)

Kopp, M.B., Bryant, A. *Geriatrics and the Law*. Springer Publisher Co. New York, NY

Schulz, J.H. *The Economics of Aging*. 4th Ed. Auburn House Publishing Co. Cover, MA

Pratt, H. *Gray Agendas: Interest Groups and Public Pensions in Canada, Britain and the U.S*. University of Michigan Press, Ann Arbor, MI (1990)

Stone, R. *"Defining Family Caregivers of the Elderly: Implication for Research and Public Policy"* The Gerontologist, Vol 3/No. 6 (1991)

Brody, B. *Wholehearted and Halfhearted Care: National Policies vs. Individual Choice* Spicher, Stuart F.

Dordrecht, H. *Ethical Dimensions of Geriatric Care* D. Reidel Publishing Co.

Carstensen, L. and Edelstein, B.A. *Handbook of Clinical Gerontology*. Bergaman Press Offices. Elmsford, NY

Unit 3 - Chapter 2

A View From the Top

The human condition has incredible resilience, rehabilitative powers and a vast supply of recuperative abilities. Those who work in the health care field are often struck with the wonder of life and its ability to sustain itself even in the most debilitated and traumatized state. From the moment a child is brought into the world until the very last breath is taken, the miracle of existence is ever-present. Understanding health and physical decline and all its complications is an essential part of being a caregiver.

As life begins to dwindle, the hope and desires of the individual change. The focus turns to leaving behind wonderful memories, legacies, momentos for future generations. Those in a position to provide care and comfort for those who need it can't possibly know the feeling of reaching the end of one's lifeline.

How do we administer to those who look to us for support and compassion when our own perceptions of life and death are in direct opposition?

One of the greatest joys of my career has been the relationships I have formed with my elderly clients. They have worlds of experience and wisdom to share, curiosity about what lies ahead and a comforting message for posterity. "Take care of yourself...you don't appreciate good health until it is gone!"

It is not often that we ask our clients what it is that they truly want for themselves. Maybe there is a fear among all of us that wewon't be able to provide whatever it is, or that it may be discomforting to realize our abilities are limited. In most cases, that which is most often requested is intangible, which forsome is more difficult than giving a pain medicine or initiating CPR.

The ansers to the question "What do you want now that your life is drawing to a close?" are universal. The names and the circumstances are different, but the response is the same. I asked hundreds of elderly folks that very question and honestly, wasn't surprised even once. Here are some of the answers:

"I want to be at home, with my family, not hooked up to machines."

"Just let me die with dignity...no machines!"

"When I can't take care of myself any longer, I want to go to a real nice nursing home, if I can afford it."

"Don't prolong the dying...just keep me comfortable."

These expressions are very much a part of a culture who believe that technology is for the young, not the old. They want to leave something behind for their children and their grandchildren and know that isn't possible if they spend it all on health care for themselves. This segment of the population is no longer making economic contributions, yet are hoping that their lifetime of investments will see them through their final years. While physical abilities, independence and support systems are diminishing, medical expenses and need for assistance is increasing. "We will lose control over our pocketbooks and our bladders, as well as all other major circumstances in our lives, including where to live, with whom to associate, what to do and what to eat." (Battin, 1987) There is no recovery from these circumstances, and though there are periods of stabilization, circumstances will continue to deteriorate until death occurs.

Hospitilization becomes a very real fear for many elderly. The issues are not only fear of not ever coming home, but also the isolation, feelings of abandonment and undue suffering which are looming possibilities. Though our goals are to keep individuals at home and healthy, many elderly find themselves in the hospital for exacerbations of chronic illness, such as heart diseasem or pulmonary congestion, or for onset of sudden illness such as stroke or bowel obstruction. We, who try so diligently to 'fix and cure' often completely miss the deepest pain, that of loneliness and anxiety. In the descriptions of hospitalizations I received, the following were frequent comments;

"I had to wait a long time for anyone to answer my light. I was very angry."

"They put me through some tests which were very painful, and they forgot to cover me up when they were done."

"The bill I got from the hospital was outrageous. I didn't know they would charge me for keeping me up all night!"

"I waited for several hours in the Emergency Room while they were getting my room ready. I thought I would get sicker if I stayed there any longer."

The positive responses were usually focused at a special individual, usually a nurse, who took the time to listen, show concern and 'make all the difference.'

"I remember the nurse who had to call three of my doctors just so that I could get a pain shot."

"I didn't know nurses need to know so much about those machines. I'm glad mine did."

"One of my nurses planted a kiss on my forehead when she thought I was sleeping."

"I'll never forget the nurse who stayed with me in the Intensive Care Unit. She held my hand and explained everything to me."

Despite the availability of hundreds of programs, certifications and specialty classes in the field of gerontology, there are few too many nurses and other health care professionals prepared to handle the issues related to the compromised older adult. For many, the terms geriatrician or geriatric specialist are unknown. This population of individuals trusted their family doctor to care for all their needs, unaware of the specialty which developed specifically for them.

The generation of elders today are the pioneers of a relatively unexplored frontier, demanding the creation and development of innovative, resourceful, and cost-effective services for every facet of the aging process. Those polled in the survey were asked about expenditures and the answers were not surprising. For those with advanced disease, requiring either 24 hr. care at home, or in long term residential care, maintaining health with frequent Doctor's office visits and medication varies from as low as $50.00/mo. to as high as $400.00/mo. depending on the type of insurance, and co-payments required.

Although only 5% of the aged are residing in long term care facilities, a much greater percentage are frequenting the emergency departments and the hospital. Frustration levels run high, not just on the part of the staff as they modify the aggressive approach most younger patients require, but also on the part of the elder patient, who would rather not be in the hospital, victims of families' wishes to 'do everything' to prolong life, despite the diminishing quality. Inappropriate expectations are a primary source for confusion on the part of all parties involved. When asked about the causes for frustration with the health care system, the responses were varied;

"I went along with what what my Dr. suggested, even though I didn't think it was such a good idea."

"I was shocked how expenses had increased since the last time I was in the hospital."

"My family wants me to be around awhile longer...but I'm really ready to go."

"The forms are so confusing; I don't know how they expect a person to be able to fill these out!"

Despite the thousands of organizations that have evolved based on the needs of the elderly, the demand is still high. Consulting services which assist with housing arrangements, placement issues and home care services are overwhelmed with calls by distraught relatives for immediate answers to elder dilemmas. Though many of the problems are typical in nature, each individual's unique circumstances challenge all of us for creative, tailor-made solutions. Education, experience and feedback assure appropriate management for the frail and impaired patient.

Many elders have become politically active, sending the message to those in pwer to consider the plight of the elderly, on fixed incomes, with rising expenses and diminishing resources. Because of the efforts of concerned legislators and lobbyists, our government has looked at issues of discrimination against the elderly and enacted laws on their behalf. The economic needs of the elderly are for lower taxes, fair prices, affordable medicine and better insurance coverage. There still exists policies which ignore the needs of certain age groups or charge outrageous premiums based on risk factors and delining health. What is it that these people would like to tell our President?

"Better long term care insurance."

"Reduce overall coverage."

"Better Social Security for all, including the next generation."

"Leave those with private insurance alone."

It is easy to empathize with those who have complex medical problems and see very little hope for stability ever again. Though society has come a long way in the development of programs and services for the elderly, it will be impossible to ever stay ahead of the demand. If there is anything which is at all responsible for the state of health and services available, it has been the creation of comprehensive medical plans by the insurance industry. Even mediocre coverage is skufficient when health is good, requiring routine check-ups and minor procedures to remain active, i.e. knee replacements, cataract surgery. The best coverage is a tremendous relief to families when ctastrophic illness threatens to deplete the value of the individual's lifetime estate.

When questioned about positive or negative experiences with the health care industry, the answers were related to the benefits and difficulties with Medicare, private insurance and the issues related to filing claims.

For a vast majority of elderly, government supplemented insurance is the only way that health care is affordable. With proper planning, individual savings and investments supplement the percent which is not covered by other types of plans. Projected figures for 1995 indicate that Medicare will serve nearly 37 million peopoe, costing approximately $156 billion. Two-thirds will be spend on hospital bills, the other one-third on non-hospital costs, such as skilled nursing facilities and home health services.

Some quotable responses regarding today's insurance coverage:

"I consider myself fortunate to have Medicare plus private insruance to take care of me if something happens."

"Even after 5 by-pass surgeries, I am still covered by my insurance!"

"My private insurance covered all my tests and surgery without excessive paperwork."

"The uncertainty about coverage after the allowed number of days in the hospital is not good. What if you're still sick?"

It is unlikely that coverage or reimbursement will ever improve from current standards. The sheer numbers of people who will require high levels of health care in the next several decades will deplete the money available. Extraordinary financial planning for the future will be essential.

Many studies have looked at the client's perception of health care. Despite grave illness, severe pain, and disability, clients find positive experiences in the hospital housekeeper may say one nurse, physician, even a special housekeeper may say or do something which alleviates the suffering, if only for a short period of time. Humans can endure massive amounts of pain and deterioration and still manage to smile at a friendly face or a kind word. Even when the task or procedure to be done is quite uncomfortable, i.e., starting an IV, or changing a dressing, etc., it is not unusual to hear a quiet 'thank you, nurse,' in reply. One moment of gratitude can be worth a thousand days of frustration and exhaustion.

What is it that clients want from us? Here are some challenging requests:

"To take care of all my needs...."

"To keep me healthy and help me take care of myself for as long as possible."

"To be treated with caring, compassion, and understanding."

"Efficiency, honesty, and kindness."

Are these realistic concerns? When you leave the academic world, do you learn the real value of life? Are these realistic concerns? When you leave the academic world, do you learn the real value of life? Are these meaningful expectations?

The resounding answer to all of these is "Absolutely!" Our call as health care professionals requires more than any of us ever expected, but not asmuch as we find strength to provide when we are called upon. The needs are escalating; the highest level of quality is expected.

A recent article in a national news publication depicted life in a nursing home from the view point of a cognitively aware individual. Her tale described the monotonous, depersonalized, generic life of someone in an institution. She openly mourned the loss of privacy and freedom and being given the dignity she so well-deserved. For those who have lost the capacity to enjoy their surroundings and look forward to the dawning of each new day, life is not so bad. For themost part, basic needs are met, with the hope that feeling loved and understood is somehow still felt. But for those who long for the symphony, the smell of burning leaves in the fall, and the sound of the church choir on Christmas morning, life becomes a mierably, lonely esistence. Even when family is involved and visit frequently, the hours drag on, marked by meals, bowel movements and medications.

The most difficult part of working and living in an institution is the realization that we have so little control over our lives, especially as the birthdays are marked by decades. Healthy older adults have traumatic accidents, frail elderly women, clinging to independence, fall over the pet cat and break hips and wrists, 97year old men who smoke cigars and enjoy back and eggs for breakfast long for heaven and a reunion with loved ones who have gone before them, and yet they wake up every day, wondering how much longer before their purpose on earth is complete. Life is not always a by-product of one's behavior. Moreover, it is a unique hand which is dealt and must be played until the last card is gone.

Control over life and death may be an option in the next century. The discussion of an individual's right to choose death is often heated, with both sides arguing about the sanctity of life with dignity. Though scientists from the 1900's couldn't predict the level of technology that would be developed, even our grandparents knew that life would be extended far beyond the bounds of their own lives.

"I figured I wouldn't live to be 60 and I'm almost 84. It feels like borrowed time for the last 24 hears."

"I thank God everyday for blessing me with all the years I have enjoyed."

"I was diagnosed with cancer 15 years ago. I can't believe I am still living."

"As long as my mind is OK, I don't mind living even longer."

Though it is a hard debate to win, institutionalizaiton has its rewards. Even though the prospect seems grim for most, the alternative could be much worse. There are many who join the ranks of those in residential housing who hae lost everyone and almost everything. Their struggles to hold onto their homes and their fortunes are meager compared to their desire not to die wihtout someone there. So often, people enter long term care facilites malnourished, depressed and physically debilitated. They are burdened by negative circumstances, knowing that being surrounded by even strangers is better than being alone.

The other side of long term care is the challenge it creates for the caregivers. Not only is it one of the most challenging types of work, it is physically and mentally exhausting, working with those who may drool while eating, are surrounded by unpleasant odors which they can no longer manage and cry out for help despite valiant efforts to provide dignity and comfort. There's something rewarding about sharing oneself with these individuals, something which responds to a need deep within, to care and keep caring because it just feels right. There are precious smiles and hands squeezed which let you know you've touched a life whose inner light is still flickering. You walk away knowing that you've made a difference, if even in the smallest way and you respect those whose wisdom has come with time.

Index

A
AARP 96
Abandonment 221
Abdomen 75, 102
Absenteeism 45
Abuse 89
    Alcohol 90
    Chemical 201
Actinic keratoses 105
Activities 88
Adaptive devices 227
Adaptive equipment 81
ADL 124, 131, 143, 229
Adult protective services 251
    Funding 251
Advance directives 52, 180
Advanced decision making 175
Aging 6, 22
Aging process 99
Agitation 215
Aid to Dependent Families 10
Airway resistance 190
Albumin 116
Alcohol 24, 124, 168, 204
Alcoholism 160
Allergic reaction 71, 74
Allergies 71, 74, 230
Alveoli 101
Alzheimer's disease 97, 159, 248
Alzheimers Disease 153
Am Assoc of Retired Persons (AARP) 251
Am Business Collaboration/Quality Depend Care 45
Amphetamines 155
Anemia 161, 166, 197
Aneurysm 196
Aneurysms 187
Angina 69, 187-188
Anorectic drugs 155
Anorexia 169
Anoxia 190
Antibiotics 213
Anticoagulants 196
Anxiety 134, 206
    Treatment of 135
Apathy 164, 197
Appendicitis 162, 194
Appetite 75, 130
Apraxia 165
Arterial narrowing 100
Arthritis 23-25, 77, 104
Aspirin 71
Assessment 4, 88, 99, 123, 131, 146, 231
Medicare 222
Assisted living 55
Assisted living centers 14
Assisted Living Facility 55
Assistive devices 87
Asthma 76, 190, 230
Atherocsclerosis 209
Atrophic 26
Atrophic vaginitis 103
Atrophy 100
Attentional deficit 167
Auscultation 101
Autoimmune disorders 198
Autonomy 64

B
B12 197
Baby boomers 6
Back injury 77
Bad blood 76
BADLs 80-81
Balance 104, 164
Barthel Index 80
Bathing 81
Beck Depression Scale 88
Bentyl 194
Bioethicists 178
Biofeedback 227
Bipolar 231
Bipolar disorder 130
Bipolar disorders 147
Bladder infection 76
Bloating 169, 209
Blood pressure 155, 188
    Control 51
Blood sugar 105, 232
Blook chemistries 105
Bowel movements 75
Bowel obstruction 193
Bowel sounds 102
Bowels 75
Bradycardia 188-189
Breast exam 26
Breath 76
Bronchitis 153
BUN 215
By-pass grafting 33

C
Cachexia 153
Caffeine 29
Calcium 29, 106
Calcium channel blockers 214
Cancer 25, 78, 230
Carcinomas 198

Cardiac conditions
    Acute 186
Cardiac output 101
Cardio-respiratory distress 167
Cardiomyopathy 161
Cardiopulmonary 166, 229
Cardiopulmonary impairment 230
Cardiovascular 72, 101
Cardiovascular disease 24
Caregiver 236
Caregivers 57
Case management 55
Cataracts 23, 230
Catastrophic illness 91
Cellular immune function 211
Centers for Disease Control 192
Cerebral neoplasms 166
Cerebrovascular Accident 178
Certified Nurse Aide 58
Cherry hemangiomas 105
Chest 101
    Expendability 101
Chest pain 69
Chief Executive Officers 46
Cholecystitis 162
Cholesterol 153
Cholesterol levels 105
Chronic conditions 25
Chronic illness 184
Chronic obstructive bronchitis 190
Chronicity 24
Cilia 101
Cirrhosis 161
Clostridium difficile 216
CNS infection 166
Cognitive assessment 67
Cognitive impairment 212
Collagen wound packing 214
Collateral source 79
Colon
    Irritable 150
Colon cancer 75
Colonoscopy 75
Colostomy 81
Combativeness 65
Commission on Accreditation for Home Care 58
Compensatory mechanisms 79
Compliance 70
confusion 65, 69, 124, 130
Congestive heart failure 188
Congestive heart failure (CHF) 187
Conjunctivitis 100
Constipation 28, 75, 194, 209
Continence 81
COPD 190

Coronary artery disease 2
Coronary artery disease (CAD) 187
Coronary bypass grafting 51
Coronary heart disease 184
Cough 192
Cranial nerve 104
Crime 156
Crohn's disease 193
Cystoceles 195

D

Daily living
    Dressing 54
    Toileting 54
Day Care 43, 222
Death 169
Debilitation 40
Debridement 214
Decreased body mass 215
decreased consciousness 153
Dehiscence 209
Dehydration 193, 197, 206
Delirium 143, 167, 211
Dementia 58, 141, 143, 153, 231
Demographics
    Volunteers 46
Dentition 28
Depappilation 100
Department of Health 58
Department of Health and Human Services 176
Dependence 64
Dependency 122
Dependency ratio 6
Depressed 77
Depression 25, 65, 128-129, 131, 143, 153, 160, 162
    Labs 131
    Life-Review 129
    Masked 129
    Somatic 129
    Therapy for 131
    Treatment of 133
Dept. of Housing & Urban Development 261
Diabetes 23, 187, 206, 214
Diabetes Mellitus 184, 198
Dialysis 222
Diastolic 101
Dietary therapy 44
Digestive disorders 153
Dignity 71
Disability 55
Disability insurance 241
Discharge 217
Disorientation 167

Distension 206
Diurectics 33
Diuretic 116
Diuretics 214
Diverticular disease 193
Dividends 12
Division of Aging 96
Dizziness 228
Do Not Resuscitate (DNR) 178
Drowsiness 91
Dry mouth 100
Durable Power of Attorney for Health Care 180
Dysarthria 196
Dysfunctional behavior 65
Dysphagia 169
Dysphoria 130
Dyspnea 223
Dysrhythmias 188
Dysthymia 130
Dysuria 196

E
Ears 100
Eccentricity 152
ECHO 56
ECOMAP
    Holman 125
Ectropion 100
Education 41, 52, 87
EENT 229
EEOC 9
Elder Housing Cottage Opportunity 56
Elderhostel 41, 96
Elderly
    Treatment 179
Elderly Cottage Housing Options (ECHO) 14
Electrolyte balance 205
Electrolyte imbalance 188
Electrolytes 215
Emboli 196
Emergencies 52
Emergency 156
Emergency department 204
Emphysema 153, 191
End of life 52, 174
Endocarditis 162
Endocrine 72, 229
Endocrine disorders 167, 214
Entropion 100
Equilibrium 187, 221
Erikson 123
Estrogen 28, 78
Ethanol abuse 166
Ethical Dilemmas 174

Excitement 155
Exercise 51, 227
    Aerobics 51
Exudates 100
Eyes 76, 99
    Cataracts 2

F
Falls 69, 203-204
Family Support Act 241
Family Support Act of 1992 250
Fat deposits 216
Fatigue 69, 130, 164
Fecal impaction 206
Federal Council on Aging 257
Fever 192, 195
Fiber 29
Financial planning 91
Fixed income 3
Flu 72
Folat deficiency 161
Folate deficiency 166
Folic acid deficiency 197
Fracture 51
Fractures 28
Fraility 149
Frequency 196
Friction 212
Functional ability 24
Functional assessment 67, 79

G
Gait 104, 227
Gallbladder 75
Gastrectomy 153
Gastritis 161
Gastrointestinal 72, 209
Gastrointestinal bleeding 154
Gastrointestinal disorders 192
Gastrointestinal System 102, 229
Gatekeepers 55
Generalized infection 166
Genitourinary 72, 229
Genitourinary disorders 194
Genitourinary/gynecologic 231
Genogram
    Mcgoldrick & Ferson 125
Geographic characteristics 34
Geriatric Depression Scale 88, 95
Geriatric Psychiatric Assesment 127
Gero-psychiatric 30
Gingivitis 100
Glaucoma 230
Glomerular tufts 195
Gray Panthers 253
Gynecologic exam 26

H

Hallucinations 215
Hamilton Depression Scale 88
Hardiness 149
Havighurst 123
Head injury 204
Headache 187, 228
Health Care Finance Administration (HCFA) 242
Health History Form 73
Health insurance 91
Health promotion 25, 51
Health promotion programs 65
Hearing 76, 150
    Deficits 70
    Loss 2, 140
Hearing impairment 23, 25
Heart disease 23
Heartburn 75
Helplessness 122, 221
Hematologic/malignant disorders 197
Hemodialysis 209
Hemoptysis 192
Hemorrhage 196
Hemorrhagic stroke 196
Hepatitis 75, 230
Hepatitis B vaccine 246
Hernia 230
Herpes zoster 216
HIV/AIDS 163
Holistic 4, 222
Home health aides 57
Homemaker 57
Hopelessness 221
Hormonal changes 26
Hospice 63, 237
Hospice programs 176
Hospital discharge 222
Hospitalization 71, 73, 150, 185
Housing 13
Huntington's Chorea 165, 167
Hydrochloric acid 192
Hygiene 54
Hypercalcemia 166
Hypercapnia 190
Hyperkalemia 157, 205
Hyperlipidemia 161
Hypertension 23, 25, 116, 131, 184, 187
Hyperthyroidism 166, 206
Hypertrophy 209
Hyperuricemia 161
Hypoalbuminemia 211
Hypoglycemia 161, 166
Hypokalemia 116, 189, 205
Hyponatremia 205
Hypoplasia 198
Hypotension 209

Hypothermia 189, 208
Hypothyroidism 106, 116, 166
Hypovolemia 209
Hypoxia 166, 211
Hysterectomy 77

I

IADL 83, 85, 124, 131, 143
IADLs 81
Iatrogenesis 150-151, 212
Ileum 193
Illness 73
Immobility 150, 212
Immune deficiency 151
Immunizations 72, 75
Immunodeficiencies 198
Impecunity 150
Impotence 151
Inanition 150
Income 10
    Median 10
    Poverty 10
Incontinence 58, 69, 150
    Products 81
Independence 64-65
    Loss of 221
Indigestion 75
Inefficient micturition 195
Infection 150, 165
Inferior MI 189
Influenza 216
Injury 214
Insomnia 91, 151, 155, 160, 215
Instability 150
Institutionalization 214
Instrumental Activities of Daily Living 81
Integumentary 228
Integumentary System 105
Intellectual impairment 150
Interactions 69
Intercourse 103
Intestinal blockage 169
Intracranial hemorrhage 197
Intracranial pressure 189
Involutional melancholia 30
Ionotropics 33
Ischemia 187
Ischemic colitis 193
Isolated systolic hypertension 186
Isolation 150, 152
Isoniazid 192

J

Jacob-Cruetzfeld's disease 167
Joint pain 77
Joint replacement 51
Judgement 64, 159

K
Katz Index of Activities of Daily Living 80
Kidney stone 76
Kidneys 102
Korsakoff's psychosis 166
Kyphosis 101, 104

L
Laboratory tests 67
Lawton Scale 80
Laxatives 71
Lean body mass 161
Lentigines 105
Life sustaining 235
Lightheadedness 189
Lipase activity 193
Lithium 154
Liver failure 166
Living Wills 181
Loneliness 211
Loss 123
Loss of spouse 64
Losses 64
    Cognitive decline 4
    Functional decline 4
    Health 4
    Independence 4
Lotion/cream 71
Lymphocytopenia 211
Lymphoid depletion 198

M
Macular degeneration 230
Magnesium 153
Major Affective Disorders 128
Malignancies 194, 198
Malignant disease 28
Malnutrition 150, 152-153, 164, 190, 206
Mammogram 78
Mandatory policy 40
Mannitol 157
Mantoux testing 192
Mass lesions 167
MCFU 259
McMasters Program 41
Medicaid 13, 73, 241
Medicare 13, 73, 241, 243, 245
Medication 71, 74, 83
Medication toxicity 215
Medications 214
Memory impairment 167
Memory loss 97
Meningitis 162
Menopause 77
Mental Health 29, 90, 122
Mental status assessment 97
Mental Status Examination 128

Mentally impaired 58
Metabolic disease 167
Metastatic carcinomas 154
Methycillin resistant staphylococcal aureus 216
MMSE 143
    Folstein 126
Mobility 43, 80, 227
Mood disorders 129
Morbidity 55, 185
Mortality 185
Motor vehicle accidents 203
Mouth 100
Multi-disciplinary 25
Multiple chronic diseases 69
Muscle retraining 227
Muscle strengthening 87
Musculoskeletal 72, 228
Musculoskeletal System 104
Mycobacterium tuberculosis 192
Myocardial infarction 187
Myoglobin 157
Myxedema 189

N
Nail fungus 104
NAOWES 254
Narcotics 206
Nasogastric tubes 191
National Council of Senior Citizens 253
National Council on Aging, Inc. 254
National Institute on Aging 22
Nausea 187
NCRA 254
Needs assessment 127
Nervous 72, 77
Neurochemical changes 142
Neurogenic lesions 165
Neurologic 228
Neurologic damage 153
Neurologic disorders 196
Neurologic dysfunction 126
Neurological System 104
NIAD 254
NICLC 254
Night sweats 77, 192
NIHPOA 254
NISC 254
NISH 254
Nitrogen levels 169
Nocturia 102
Noncompliance 65
Nose 100
Nosocomial infection 216
Nosocomial infections 186
Nursing home 58

Nursing homes 14
Nursing intervention 146
Nutrition 26, 152
Nutritional anemia 153
Nutritional disorders 25
NVOILA 254

O
OARS 80, 83, 88
OARS Social Resource Scale 92
OASIS 96
Obesity 154-155
OBRA 58
Obstruction 194
Occlusive dressing 214
Occupational therapy 63
Octogenarians 6, 9
Oculomotor nerve 104
Older American's Act 242
Older Americans' Act 255
Older Women's League 258
Omnibus Budget Reconcilliation Act 176
Omnibus Reconciliation Act 255
Omnibus Reconcilliation Act 241
Onchymycosis 104
Opportunistic infection 164
Optimal health 4
Organic brain syndrome 167
Orthopedic 23, 28
Osteomalacia 153
Osteoporosis 25, 28-29, 104
    Primary 28
    Secondary 28
Osteoporotic 2
Ostomy 230
Outreach programs 52
Oxygen saturation 208

P
Pacemaker 33
Pain 160
Palpation 101
Pap smear 26, 78
Papilledema 100
Paranoia 139-140, 165
Paraphrenia 139
Parkinson's diesease 167
Parkinson's Disease 165
Parlysis 196
Peck 123
Pelvic 26
Pensions 12
Pepsin 192
Perception 64, 159
Peripheral edema 188
Peripheral neuropathy 204
Peripheral vascular disease 189

Peritonitis 194
Personality
    Disorders 136-138
    Styles 136
Physical Exam Form 106
Physical examination 67
Physical therapy 44, 63, 87
Pick's disease 167
Platelet count 164
Pnemonia 164
Pneumococcal pneumonias 191
Pneumococcal/Influenza 246
Pneumonia 72, 191, 206, 216, 230
Polycythemia 197
Polypharmacy 150, 200
Polyps 75
Poor oxygenation 188
Post-anesthesia reaction 168
Post-anesthesia symptoms 166
Postmenopausal 28
Postural hypotension 101
Postural instability 204
Potassium 116, 153
Poverty 10, 150, 152
Power of Attorney 181
Power of Attorney in Fact 180
Preretirement planning 52
Presbycusis 100, 206
Presbyopia 206
Pressure
    Normal 166
Pressure ulcers 186
    Grades 213
    Treatment 213
Productivity 45
Proprioception 204
Prostate 76
Prostate screening antigen (PSA) 105
Prostatism 195
Protein-energy malnutrition (PEM) 210
Proxy 181
Depression 130
Psychiatric 77
Psychiatric assessment 127
Psychiatric disorders 127
Psychoactive medications 201
Psychodynamic assessment 127
Psychological disorders 214
Psychomotor 129
Psychomotr activity 167
Psychosocial 4, 125, 160, 201
    Stressors 151
Psychosocial Assessment 67, 87
Psychosocial distress 168
Ptyalin 192
Pubic hair 103

Pulmonary 72
Pupil response 228
Q
Quality of life 67
R
Radiation 222
Receptor antagonists 194
Reconciliation 170
Recreation 44
Rectum 102
Regional Coordinating Council/Older Americans 41
Rehabilitation 54
Reimbursement 235
Renal failure 154, 166, 187, 194
Renal perfusion 157
Renal System 102
Reproductive System 103
Resident Bill of Rights 58
Resources 40
Respiratory
    Distress 190
Respiratory disorders 190
Respite for caregiver 44
Restorative 54
Retirees 9
Retirement 9, 123
Retirement Centers 14
Rhabdomyolysis 157
Risk factors 156
S
Sandwich Generation 53
Schizophrenia 139, 231
Scurvy 153
Sebaceous glands 105
Seborrheic keratoses 105
Secretions 101
Seisure 228
Seizure 205
Self-determination 175
Self-neglect 162
Senior Centers 42
Senior Citizen's Bill of Rights 242
Senior Corp of Retired Executives (SCORE) 41
Senses
    Vibration 105
Sensory 72
Serum albumin 153
Sexual function 161
Sexual relations 76
Sexual transmission 163
Shearing 212
Short Blessed Test of Orientation Memory Conc 98

Sigmoidoscopy 75
Silver segment 33
Sinusitis 23
Skilled nursing facilities 176
Skilled Nursing Facility 243
Skin 72, 76, 105
Skin ulcers 162
Sleep
    Apnea 91
    Disturbance 129
Sleep disorders 90
Smoking 71, 74, 187
Social isolation 211, 221
Social Security 12
Socialization 44
Socioeconomic 28
Speech therapy 87
SPMSQ 126
Spouse 57
Sputum culture 192
Sr. Citizens Transportation Assist Program 43
Steroids 154
Stomach 75
Stress incontinence 26
Stroke 28, 166, 196
Subarachnoid space 196
Subdural hematoma 166
Sudden death 187
Suicide 131-132
    Assessment 132
Sundowning 206
Surgery 74
Surrogate 91
Swallowing
    Difficulties 153
Swelling 76
Syncope 187, 204
Syphilis 76
Systolic 101
T
T-cell function 198
Tachycardias 155
Temperature 206
Tetanus 72
The Patient Self-Determination Act 176
Therapy 146
Thermal injuries 203
Thrombi 196
Thrombotic stroke 196
Thymic atrophy 198
Thyroid 77
Thyroid disease 214
TIA 204
Tinnitus 23

Title I-Declaration of Objective 256
Title II - Administration on Aging 257
Title III 257
Title IIIB - Supportive Services 257
Title IV - Training & Research 258
Title V - Sr Community Service Employment Pro 258
Title VI - Grants to Native Americans 258
Total body water 161
Toxic substances 168
Toxicity 69
Tranquilizers 154
Transient ischemic attach (TIA) 187
Transient ischemic attacks (TIA) 196
Transition 53
Transportation 43
Trauma 51, 168, 197
Tremor 104, 228
Tremors 164
Tubercle bacilli 192
Tuberculosis 162, 191

U
Ulcer 75
Ulcerative colitis 193
Ultrasound 227
Unconsciousness 174
Urinalysis 105
Urinary Tract 102
Urinary tract infection 162
Urinary tract infection (UTI) 195
Urinate 76
Urine culture 215
Urosepsis 169
Urostomy 81
US Commission on Civil Rights 9
Uterine prolapse 26
UTI 206, 215

V
Vagina 26, 78
Varicosities 23
Vascularization 100
Vasculitis 166
Vasodilators 33
Vegetative state 174
Vertigo 187
Vial of Life 52
Vision 76, 150
    Deficits 70
Visual impairment 25, 223
Vit B12 166, 206
Vit C 213
Vitamin 71
Vitamin B6 153
Vitamin D 153
Vitamin deficiency 161

Vitamins 106
Voice 76
Volunteers 46
Vomiting 187
Vulva 26

W
Wages 12
Weakness 70, 186
Weight 28
Weight loss 192
Weight training 51
Wet lung sounds 188
Wills 52

X
Xerosis 105

Y
Yellow jaundice 75
YMCA 51

Z
Zantac 194
Zero Population Growth 6
Zero Population Growth (ZPG) 240